2014

RECOVER QUICKLY FROM SURGERY

The Essential Guide for Reducing Your
Pain, Swelling and Recovery Time

*To our loving parents, who believe in us and
to all the innovators in complementary medicine
who have inspired this work.*

DISCLAIMER

This information is not intended to treat, diagnose, cure or prevent any disease and has not been evaluated by the Food and Drug Administration. Rather, it is provided for educational purposes only. Please be aware that this information is provided to supplement the care provided by your physician. It is neither intended nor implied to be a substitute for professional medical advice or treatment, nor is it meant to discourage the reader from obtaining advice from his or her physician. Any dietary or lifestyle change should be undertaken only with the approval and supervision of your physician. If you have any questions regarding the information contained in this book, please review and discuss the options herein with your surgeon and primary physician, especially if you have an unusual medical condition or other constraint that might conflict with some or all of the information in this book. If you are pregnant, nursing, have cancer or currently are using prescription medications, you should also consult with your physician before making any dietary or lifestyle changes proposed herein.

Published by
PANHARMONIC PRESS
1725 State Street B, Santa Barbara, CA 93101

Ordering Information:
Quantity sales. Special discounts are available on quantity purchases by corporations, associations, and others. For details, contact the publisher at the address above. Orders by U.S. trade bookstores and wholesalers. Please contact PanHarmonic Press @ www.panharmonicpress.com

Book and cover design by Jenny VanSeters, Santa Barbara, CA
Printed in the United States of America

ISBN 13 NUMBER 978-0-9898821-0-1
Library of Congress Control Number: 2013918712

The Complete Guide For Pre and Post Surgery
Preparation Using Clinically-Tested Natural Protocols
That Can Accelerate Your Recovery

RECOVER QUICKLY FROM SURGERY

The Essential Guide for Reducing Your Pain, Swelling, and Recovery Time

by Dr. Valerie Girard

with Michelle K. Gysan

PANHARMONIC PRESS ● SANTA BARBARA, CA

PRAISE FOR RECOVER QUICKLY FROM SURGERY

Dr. Girard's approach in assisting patients with healing from surgery is highly effective and easy for everyone. Her book's protocols not only helped me return to work within a week after my knee surgery, but can make a difference in improving your health and longevity over a lifetime.
—DR. STEVE SHERWIN

For three weeks prior to, and three weeks following, a cosmetic surgery procedure, I strictly followed Dr. Girard's regimen of the Anti-Inflammation Diet plus nutritional and homeopathic supplements, and followed up with several cold laser treatments* at the suture sites. (This regime was in fact almost exactly the same as recommended by my highly regarded surgeon.) Although I am fair-skinned and have a very low clotting factor, predisposing me to bruise easily, I experienced only minimal post-surgical bruising and inflammation, and no pain. Everyone, including staff at my surgeon's office, was astonished at my super-quick recovery. I had imagined that I would be recuperating and hiding out for weeks following the surgery. Instead, less than two days later I was walking for 30 minutes, four days later I was eating out in restaurants, and just 10 days post-surgery I received the OK to return to my aerobics routine. I couldn't have asked for a better, quicker recovery.
—LAURIE D.

I have had three joint replacement surgeries in the last three years involving a shoulder, a knee, and a hip. Before and after each surgery, Dr. Valerie Girard provided me with supplements to reduce inflammation, others to hasten the healing process, along with chiropractic treatments, advice on nutrition, general support with her holistic approach to well-being, and her caring attitude. Dr. Girard was very instrumental in my rapid recovery from these surgeries. I would highly recommend her treatments for anyone facing health issues, including surgery.
—P. GREGORY

I followed Dr Girard's pre surgery diet protocol for a month prior to my complete knee replacement surgery to reduce any inflammation in my body. Following the surgery I continued with diet, physical therapy and laser treatments given by Dr Girard. I was able to , in just a few weeks, reduce the pain medication to a minimum. In 10 weeks I was off pain medication and able to walk a mile a day. At this point my surgeon said, after watching me walk, said " You are my Poster boy and I don't need to see you for a year". I am 83 and since then I have been walking 2 miles a day plus mountain hikes on the weekend.
—EDWARD G.

CONTENTS

Introduction: The Silver Lining 9

    Who Should Read This Book 9

    From My Experience 10

    You Can Participate in Your Surgery's Success 11

    The Power of Integrative Medicine 12

    Who Uses Integrative Medicine? 13

    Why Integrative and Complementary Medicine Can
    Help You Recover Faster...14

    More Physicians Are Incorporating Natural Therapies
    with Western Medicine..15

    How This Book Will Facilitate an Easier, Faster Recovery 15

CHAPTER 1: Preparation is Key 19

    Creating Your Dynamic Health Care Team............................19

    6 Keys to Finding the Right Surgeon 20

    Interviewing Your Surgeon: Asking the Right Questions 23

    Appointing an Advocate for Your Surgery...........................26

    Becoming an Advocate for Someone Who Requires Surgery...........27

    Empower Your Surgery with Research..............................28

    This Is Your Time to Nurture Yourself 29

CHAPTER 2: Improving Your Fitness to Enhance Recovery 31

    Recovery Starts Before Surgery with Prehabilitation 32

    The Three Types of Fitness that Can Help You Recover Faster 33

CHAPTER 3: Change Your Lifestyle and Recover Quickly 41

    Research Reveals the Secrets to Healing Faster......................41

CHAPTER 4: Heal Faster with the Recover Quickly Diet..................49

    Why This Specific Diet Can Enhance Your Recovery 49

    The Recover Quickly Diet 52

CHAPTER 5: The Essential Two Drinks to Accelerate Recovery 63

CHAPTER 6: Nutritional Supplements to Expedite Your Recovery 71

The Optimum Supplement Protocol for Your Rapid Recovery 71

What Are Enzymes? 72

Homeopathy to Augment Your Healing Process 80

Protocols for Joint Surgeries 81

Quick Guide for Nutritional Supplementation 82

Food and Supplements to Avoid Before Surgery 85

CHAPTER 7: Acupuncture: Accelerate Healing, Decrease Pain **89**

Acupuncture Can Reduce Your Need for Pain Medication 90

Applying Acupressure Points 91

CHAPTER 8: Sleep To Recover **93**

Sleep: The Ultimate Recovery Tool 93

15 Causes of Insomnia. 93

Effective Natural Sleep Supplements. 97

CHAPTER 9: Prepare Emotionally for Surgery **99**

Capitalize on the Mind-Body Connection 99

The Effects of Negative Emotions on Surgery 101

Are Your Thoughts Hurting You? 101

An Emotional Clearing Technique 103

CHAPTER 10: The Body-Mind Connection and Surgery **111**

Empower Your Healing Process with Affirmations. 111

Meditation to Accelerate the Healing Process 115

Self-Generated Meditation Practices 116

Guided Meditation 116

Creative Visualization 117

Tips for Effective Creative Visualization 118

Recover Quickly Through Hypnosis 121

CHAPTER 11: Pain: What to Expect **123**

Ask Your Surgeon in Advance 124

Addiction 125

Inform Your Doctor. 125

Managing Your Pain. 126

A Plan For Pain: Non-Traditional Pain Management 127

Essential Natural Pain Supplements 128
10 Effective Pain Management Treatments.........................129

CHAPTER 12: Detoxifying From Medication **135**
11 Gentle Cleansing Options 136

CHAPTER 13: Preventing Scarring **141**
Preventing Wound Infections 141
Common Types of Scars 143
Pre-Surgery Protocols...144
Heal Your Incision, Prevent Scarring 144
Early Care for Incisions...146
Effective Scar-Reducing Therapies 146
The Psychological Factor of Scarring 148

CHAPTER 14: Summary: Key Preparation **149**
One Month Before Surgery 150
Two Weeks Before Surgery 151
Utilizing the Recover Quickly Diet...............................152
Rest and Sleep 153
The Day Before Surgery 153
What to Pack for the Hospital 155

CHAPTER 15: Practical Matters.....................................**157**
18 Steps to Prepare for Post Surgical Recovery 157

CHAPTER 16: The Day of Your Surgery **161**
Hospital Admittance: The Routine................................161
Your Hospital Stay 162
Questions for Your Surgeon After Surgery 163
Discharge from The Hospital 164
Medical Emergencies 164

CHAPTER 17: Hindsight **167**
The Power of Insight..167
The Role of Genetics 168
View Your Surgical Experience as a Catalyst.....................169

THE SILVER LINING

Every human being is the author of
his own health or disease.

—Siddhartha, the founder of Buddhism, 563-483 B.C.

The need for surgery can be alarming. It can come at an inopportune time and represent time away from family and work. The specter of pain during the recovery period can be daunting.

If you have picked up this book because you or a loved one requires surgery, this guide will augment your recovery process. Research herein provides new evidence of strategies that can shorten your recovery time, reduce pain and scarring. Armed with new clinical studies, this book will empower you to proactively participate in your healing from surgery. With this knowledge, your surgery can serve as a catalyst in making long overdue changes in your habits, lifestyle or personal outlook.

Therein lies the silver lining.

WHO SHOULD READ THIS BOOK

This book is not designed for those individuals who want to use alternative therapies *instead* of surgery. Rather, this essential guide recommends that you utilize specific natural medicine and treatments *together* with surgery and conventional medicine. Specifically, this book is tailored to those who are planning to undergo surgery and who have at least two weeks or more to prepare in advance for it. Anyone who is about to undergo surgery wants to reduce pain and heal as quickly as possible so that they can move forward in their lives. Supported by a plethora of clinical studies, this book will guide you in utilizing specific natural protocols, before and after surgery, which can accelerate your recovery time, reduce pain, swelling and promote a faster, easier recovery.

FROM MY EXPERIENCE

Like most of you reading this book, I faced the need for surgery. As a chiropractor and nutritional practitioner for nearly thirty years, I have assisted many patients in preparing for surgery. When it became evident that I needed to undergo abdominal surgery, a variety of questions and emotions arose. After consulting with several doctors, I made the decision to have the surgery. Once scheduled, I was determined to make my surgical experience as positive as possible and wanted to recover quickly so that I could resume my life and career.

Fortunately, my health issue did not require immediate attention. I had one month to prepare for my procedure. After interviewing several recommended surgeons. I weighed their suggestions and carefully chose a surgeon based on several factors outlined in this book.

With a month to prepare, I designed a protocol of specific anti-inflammatory vitamins and supplements. These included supplements that would reduce swelling as well as help detoxifying any anesthesia or drugs that might be used during my procedure. I changed my diet to exclude foods and beverages that were inflammatory and included those that would enhance and accelerate my recovery. I included treatments such as acupuncture and laser therapy in my recovery process. I also utilized effective body-mind exercises and meditation techniques that I have shared with patients and students over the years to overcome my fear and anxiety about surgery.

I was very pleased with my post-surgical results. I had little pain and didn't require prescribed pain medication. Two days later, I noted another fifty percent improvement. Within five days I was able to hike and bike with no pain. From that moment, I had no more inflammation, pain or side effects.

My surgeon agreed that I had healed faster than the average patient undergoing a similar surgery. He noted that when he made four incisions, I barely bled. There was no swelling or redness and the incisions healed within a week. In addition, over time, there was no apparent scarring. The pain I had experienced before the surgery was completely gone—to my relief. Because of the antioxidants I had taken, there were no side effects from the anesthesia.

What I had prescribed to hundreds of patients worked exceptionally well for me. Surprisingly, just a week after the surgery, I felt more empowered and healthier than I had before. Similarly, the majority of my patients who followed my prescribed regimen reported a notable reduction in pain and swelling. They often reported their physicians telling them that they had healed in half the time.

Having found almost no recent published compendium of effective natural healing protocols for surgery, I became excited to share this process with my patients and others who might benefit from this information. I want to empower others to actively participate in their recovery process and experience the same success in reducing pain and recovering quickly.

YOU CAN PARTICIPATE IN YOUR SURGERY'S SUCCESS

In writing this book, first and foremost I want to educate and empower surgical patients to contribute to the success of their own surgery. Gaining knowledge about the natural and alternative supplements, therapies and resources available is your right. Importantly, this education and awareness gives you more control and power to participate in and enhance your recovery process.

Education and Preparation Can Expedite Your Recovery

Many patients about to undergo surgery ask, "Why not leave my medical care solely to my physician? Why go beyond the common medical model to pursue natural healing practices? Isn't Western medicine the best option available? Do complementary therapies really work?"

The scope of a surgeon or physician's role usually does not include implementing the kind of health protocols outlined in this book. Thus, you might be omitting many essential measures that will reduce pain, swelling, scarring and decrease recovery time. The old adage "We don't know what we don't know" rings true here. Educating yourself about your options gives you the power to make critical choices in your own healing.

Importantly, education and awareness gives you more control and power to participate in and enhance your recovery process.

Recent studies show that the more active a patient is active in making their own healthcare decisions, the better the outcome and the lower the costs associated with the health issue. Most importantly, research suggests that the more patients are educated about their surgery, the more likely they are to experience less pain and enjoy a faster recovery. One 2003 clinical trial involving hip surgery revealed that patients who were more educated about approaching surgical procedures were significantly less anxious before surgery than patients who received a minimal education. Those who were more educated about surgical options and process, experienced *less* pain after surgery and were able to stand sooner. [1]

THE POWER OF INTEGRATIVE MEDICINE

Combining Traditional Medicine with Complementary Medicine Can Ease and Hasten Your Recovery

This guide introduces an "integrative" approach to preparing for and healing faster from your surgery. This approach utilizes *both* Western (or mainstream medicine) and complementary or natural medicine to accelerate the healing process and produce optimum results for an easier, faster surgical recovery.

Western medicine typically utilizes surgery, physical therapy and pharmaceutical drugs as its primary form of healthcare, managing health issues or injuries rather than preventing them.

Complementary or natural medicine practitioners-including chiropractors, acupuncturists, nutritionists, osteopaths and naturopaths —use nutritional supplements, physical medicine, acupuncture, nutritional counseling, exercise therapy, diet and lifestyle modification as well as 'energetic medicine' to treat the *source* of an illness or injury.

Together, traditional and complementary medicine can powerfully combine treatments or protocols to form integrative medicine where the two approaches work harmoniously together.

WHO USES INTEGRATIVE MEDICINE?

The use of integrative medicine worldwide has increased substantially over the last two decades. Europe, notably Germany, uses complementary medicine as a first line treatment before resorting to more costly medical procedures. Why? With timely implementation, integrative or complementary medicine often has fewer side effects and is much more cost effective overall. As one of the fastest growing sectors in health care, the use of herbs, natural supplements, specific dietary protocols, chiropractic care, acupuncture, nutrition based therapies, homeopathy, yoga, meditation and other various therapies are rapidly becoming integrated into modern healthcare.

Many American university hospitals, including the Mayo Clinic, Duke University, Ohio State University Medical Center, Cleveland Clinic and dozens more, are now adding centers for integrative medicine. A large volume of research and recent studies published by renowned health institutions including the National Institute of Health indicate that various forms of complementary therapies are extremely effective as pre-operative and post-operative procedures.

About 38 percent of Americans use natural or alternative therapies and approximately 50 percent worldwide in developed countries. [2]

As the industry expands, more stringent licensing and accredited educational requirements have been instituted, especially for chiropractors, acupuncturists, naturopaths and osteopaths. These practitioners are now considered primary care providers, recognized by major medical insurance companies, Medicare and Workman's Compensation. This gives the integrative medicine field more accreditation with a strong, educational focus.

WHY INTEGRATIVE AND COMPLEMENTARY MEDICINE CAN HELP YOU RECOVER FASTER

Unlike conventional medicine, which generally waits to address health problems *after* they become an issue, integrative medicine's modalities are preventative by nature. The intent of integrative medicine is to strengthen the immune system, reduce inflammation in the body and support a healthy physiology thereby reducing the risk of both acute and chronic disease. Increasingly, research is showing that inflammation and toxicity are the primary causes of disease in the body. In this context, clinical research shows that using integrative medicine effectively can accelerate recovery time and reduce pain. This is the primary reason that many hospitals are creating new divisions for research and implementation of integrative medicine.

In addition to surgery and medication, an integrative approach might include dietary changes to reduce inflammation and the use of specific nutritional supplements that have been shown to effectively assist in the recovery process. An integrative approach might promote exercise and yoga therapy to accelerate recovery time if appropriate for the patient. It advocates mind-body practices to increase healing potential and reduce stress, as well as the use of alternative therapies to reduce pain, accelerate recovery and promote lifestyle changes.

MORE PHYSICIANS ARE INCORPORATING NATURAL THERAPIES WITH WESTERN MEDICINE

This system of treating patients is emerging as individual practitioners on both sides of medicine educate themselves about available therapies, keeping their patient's best interest in mind while treating them.

Integrative medicine will function at its best if the patient seeks doctors and other practitioners who are educated about medical and alternative modalities. Over the last decade, more physicians have seen the remarkable advantages of supplementing traditional medicine with acupuncture, chiropractic, herbal and natural supplements, laser therapies and other natural treatments to augment their treatment programs.

There are many fine medical doctors who have not had any exposure to viable integrative, natural medical practices. Therefore, it is often up to the patient to seek complementary care with a natural care practitioner. This practitioner can collaborate with the surgeon about their patient's integrative care options in light of an approaching surgery.

HOW THIS BOOK WILL GUIDE YOU TO AN EASIER, FASTER RECOVERY

First and foremost I wish to educate and empower surgical patients to be able to contribute to the success of their own surgery and recovery. In gaining these insights, this book will guide you in:

1. your use of specific nutritional protocols that have been clinically known to be extremely effective in accelerating your recovery, reducing pain and minimizing scarring;

2. understanding how alternative therapies such as acupuncture,

chiropractic and the use of specific nutritional supplements are clinically proven to be effective in pain management, reducing swelling, decreasing recovery time and scarring;

3. choosing both the correct surgeon and the appropriate holistic health practitioner who will work in unison to enhance your recovery process;

4. creating an easy, delicious anti-inflammatory diet that will reduce pain and side effects incurred before and after your surgical process. (Research indicates that adherence to specific diets before, during and after surgery can expedite your recovery process.);

5. gaining a deeper understanding of the mind-body connection and how it relates to your condition, recovery, pain levels and your management of pain. The book includes specific exercises and processes that may reduce stress, calm the mind and empower healing;

6. adopting an empowering lifestyle that will greatly reduce your risk of disease, as well as promoting increased energy levels and improved health and well-being.

BY PARTICIPATING MORE IN YOUR SURGERY'S PREPARATION, IT'S WITHIN YOUR REACH TO:

- experience as little pain as possible with the least amount of medication;

- decrease swelling and pain with fewer residual symptoms as possible;

- reduce risks of infection and other complications by enhancing your immune system prior to surgery;

- achieve an improved level of health and fitness to accelerate your recovery;

- resume a normal or improved level of activity quickly;

- minimize scarring and body disfigurement;

- reduce the need for future surgeries in the same area at a later time;

- alleviate pre-surgical fear by learning relaxation techniques that are effective and beneficial before and after your surgery;

- retain the lessons learned to enhance your life after surgery and gain an increased positive outlook about life from hereafter.

There is a significant amount of research that concludes that specific body-mind therapies may enhance your health. The second half of this book introduces exercises that induce a positive mental state as well as assist in managing pain and obtaining sound sleep. These exercises will not only help you prepare for your surgery, but will be extremely useful for other emotional challenges in your life beyond your surgical experience.

Most of these benefits fall outside of the surgeon's purview. If any or all of these results appeal to you, then you are ready to play an important part in your own recovery. The first step is to educate yourself about what actions you can take to recover more quickly.

EXPECT SUCCESS

Approach your surgery with the same expectation of success that you have for other significant projects in your life. By examining your nutritional intake and diet, your current exercise routine (if any), your overall physical condition, as well as your mental and emotional attitude, you can empower your healing beyond the scope of your medical procedure. *You can begin your recovery process now by implementing any of these protocols today.*

Nothing in this book is meant to diagnose or treat your condition. You must, after reading this book, discuss the best way to implement the appropriate natural supplements and therapies with your surgeon and design a timeline and program for their use before and after surgery. Together, you and your surgeon can collaborate on tailoring a plan designed specifically for you.

PREPARATION IS KEY

By failing to prepare, you are preparing to fail.

—Benjamin Franklin

CREATE YOUR DYNAMIC HEALTH TEAM

First and foremost, it is important to choose the best surgeon possible for your condition. Second, you must locate the complementary practitioners, such as a chiropractor, acupuncturist or nutritionist that will assist you in implementing your plan to recover quickly. These natural practitioners should offer a variety of "protocols", such as herbs, nutritional supplements, diet, homeopathy, acupuncture and energetic medicine that will support your recovery.

WHAT IS A PROTOCOL?

A protocol is a series of procedures that when followed, provide a specific result. The natural protocols and suggestions outlined are meant to complement your physician's plan for your surgery by easing and accelerating your recovery process. With your doctor's guidance, choose the protocols suitable for you and your condition. The health protocols identified herein should be altered and tailored specifically for you, depending on your particular health issue, the nature of your surgery and your unique health condition and tolerances by your physician, nutritionist or other qualified holistic care practitioner who fully understands the impact nutrition and integrative medicine has on your wellness.

You may choose to have several practitioners treating you, as it is desirable to have acupuncture, massage and chiropractic care before surgery. These treatments tend to boost the resiliency of the body, increase the immune response and provide the necessary relaxation to reduce anxiety and fear you may experience about your approaching surgery. An ideal team consists of your surgeon, your anesthesiologist, other medical consultants, a complementary health care practitioner who will oversee your preparations, as well as those who will enhance your recovery, such as acupuncturists, chiropractors, osteopaths, nutritionists and naturopaths.

6 KEYS TO FINDING THE RIGHT SURGEON

It is important that you seek advice from the experts. They have spent years studying and treating others with your condition. That said, it is generally wise to gather information regarding your condition or injury from several sources. If a surgeon or physician's advice makes you feel uncertain, seek advice from another surgeon as well as one in an alternative field. There are six essential factors to consider when choosing your ideal surgeon.

1. **Acceptance of Integrative Medicine.** Ideally, the surgeon that you choose will be accepting of complementary or natural medicine to augment your healing. Be wary of the physician that discourages you from implementing complementary or natural medicine in your recovery process. True healing happens on many levels and is a cooperative effort. It requires the compliance of the patient as well as the insight of the practitioners involved. Many physicians have not been educated in the areas of nutrition and do not understand the powerful impact that natural therapies can have on your recovery.

   You may want to approach your surgeon armed with recent medical studies, research and reports in favor of the benefits of some of these protocols. Nutrition alone is a tremendously expanding field, with research supporting the use of vitamins, supplements and herbs as an addition (and sometimes alternative) to medication. More physicians are slowly integrating the use of nutrition and supplements in their practice even as cutting edge hospitals throughout the world are creating departments for integrative medicine.

Cosmetic surgeons appear to be leaders in understanding the benefits of integrative medicine. Many are encouraging their patients to use specific supplements and natural anti-inflammatory protocols known to reduce swelling and scarring, thereby increasing positive post-surgical results.

2. **Get a Second Opinion.** Do not automatically use the first doctor or surgeon recommended. If you have time, you should always consult with at least two recommended physicians. It could change the course of your life. Each one may have differing opinions about the scope and invasiveness of surgery, the risks involved and options for you to consider.

Once you decide to have surgery, interview at least two surgeons with the highest expertise in his or her field. Doing so will either give you more confidence in proceeding with your surgery or it might prompt you to further investigation. No practitioner is infallible, and sometimes that second opinion can save your life or prevent an unpleasant recovery.

3. **Feel Confident About Your Doctor.** Some physicians may seem intimidating or may not explain things in the simplest manner. Do not be shy about asking them to explain all aspects and risks of your surgery clearly to you. Ultimately, you want to feel confident about their level of attention towards your concerns and questions, as well as their overall experience and

recommendations. At the end of the consultation, you should feel that you trust them and their ability to help you.

4. **Ask Your Surgeon if There Are Alternative Surgical Procedures.** A good surgeon should discuss several options for your health issue, as well as the efficacy and risks involved with those options. Be wary if they discredit other doctors or processes without offering solid evidence. There are now several ways to perform surgeries so be sure to ask which is best for your condition. Ask if there are experts performing those alternative procedures.

5. **Get Another Opinion from a Natural Health Practitioner.** If possible, get another opinion from a natural health provider, such as a chiropractor, acupuncturist, nutritionist or osteopath. They may offer alternative options and treatments as a solution to your issue. I have known several women who have used herbs, homeopathy and supplements to shrink cysts and fibroids. Many of my patients have avoided back surgery by obtaining chiropractic care. If surgery is determined to be inevitable, then your natural health care practitioner might be able to recommend a great surgeon for your condition.

6. **Use Referral Resources.** Friends, relatives and physicians are an optimum referral source. If you know physicians that are not surgeons, ask them for referrals for the best in the field pertaining to your health issue, especially if your situation is serious. They may refer someone in another town or part of the country that is a specialist in that field.

If someone you know has had your condition, ask how they resolved their problem. Ask them how they felt about the procedures they experienced. Do they have any regrets? Ask what they would have done differently. If one of your acquaintances has used alternative medicine to heal their condition, ask them about their results. The Internet may also be a referral source for surgeons and health practitioners.

INTERVIEWING YOUR SURGEON: ASKING THE RIGHT QUESTIONS

Asking the proper questions for your procedure means receiving more thorough answers. Bring paper with you, write down as many detailed questions as possible in advance and allow room beneath each question for the physician's answers. If you are not able to listen and write down the surgeon's answers, bring someone with you who can perform that function. Read your questions before the discussion with your surgeon and add any additional questions that come to mind. The following suggested questions are listed on the Recover Quickly website. You may wish to print these out with your additional questions and include space to write the answers.

Is this surgery necessary? What are the risks and benefits? What are all of the complete surgical options?

How soon? How urgent is this surgery? By when should it be performed to be effective?

Are they aware of any natural or complementary therapies? Are they open to you exploring them?

Can your surgery be done with less invasive procedures such as laparoscopy or robotic surgery? Can your surgeon perform laparascopic or robotic surgery?

How many surgeries of this kind has your surgeon performed in the past?

What is their success rate for performing your surgery? What is the overall success rate for anyone having your surgery?

What are the predictable outcomes? What can you expect from the surgery? What are the risks and their percentages for occurrence? What are the possible side effects?

What is a typical length of recovery? Does the surgeon have any suggestions for speeding up recovery?

Is there a possibility that cancer is involved? If so, you might want to consult an oncologist who is also a surgeon. You may be asked to sign an agreement advising your surgeon of how he or she should proceed, if cancer is found.

Will your surgeon follow your wish to include natural protocols when possible?

Will he or she allow you to substitute or combine natural remedies for pain medication whenever possible?

Will he or she make every attempt to save your organs if possible?

What are the possible side effects of anesthesia? Will you require anesthesia? Will you be awake or asleep during the surgery? Does the doctor recommend a particular anesthesiologist? Should you have a separate consultation with them? Will they be present during the surgery? What is your personal risk of anesthesia complications based on your current level of health?

Will the anesthesiologist be open to using positive language during the operation? Are you allowed to bring in an audio device,

PATIENT SUCCESS STORY

A patient was considering a corneal transplant. His cornea was so misshaped that he could only see with specialized contact lenses. These contacts popped out of his eyes continually, causing him near blindness and hours wasted in finding the lenses. His well-regarded eye doctor had advised against the surgery, claiming his cornea was too thin to hold the stitches.

Discouraged, he avoided surgery and spent years in frustration and discomfort. Finally, years later, someone gave him a reference for a second opinion. He drove almost two hours to the next doctor, who ran a center specializing in eye surgery. The good news revealed a high success rate with this doctor's procedures. Encouraged, he drove back to this city to get a third opinion. This doctor, operating out of a university medical center, also offered a positive prognosis for success.

He chose the doctor from the university medical center because he felt a high rapport with the doctor and his staff. Because the stakes were high, he also followed my pre and post surgery advice, knowing that he wanted to do anything he could to insure success. Failure meant blindness in that eye.

He followed the Recover Quickly From Surgery Protocols closely. He took the suggested supplements, ate an anti-inflammatory diet, maintained a positive attitude and followed his doctor's post-surgical advice to the letter.

The result? The doctor claimed that he is the poster boy for corneal transplants.

such as an iPod or MP3 player so that you can listen to your music or guided meditations?

Are there any adverse reactions that may occur between the

medications needed for the surgery and any vitamins or medications that you are currently taking?

What tests will be needed before the surgery? Can any recent tests be substituted? Are any tests elective? What are their costs?

What are all of the potential surgical costs? If you are a cash patient, is there a cash discount?

Is your doctor a provider for your insurance? Ask the doctor to recommend which labs, anesthesiologists and radiologists are on your plan.

What is the expected recovery time? How many days will you be hospitalized? How many days of solid bed rest is required or recommended? How long before you can return to work? How long before you can engage in physical activity such as lifting, gardening or sports?

Will you need rehabilitation? Do you need physical therapy and, if so, for how long? Will you need in-home rehab or go to a rehab center? Are there home exercises that will facilitate your recovery? Can the doctor recommend an excellent rehabilitation service?

Will you need skilled nursing? If so, for how many days and for how long each day? Who will arrange the nursing care? Will you need a hospital bed, wheelchair or walker?

APPOINTING AN ADVOCATE FOR YOUR SURGERY

In some cases, you may be too weak or ill to make your own decisions. It might be difficult to even ask for nutritional supplements or special foods. In this case, it is important to have someone oversee your healing process. Ideally, they will be able to read this book and assist you in implementing some of the protocols into your healing process.

Additionally, there may be too many decisions to make regarding your care. If so, it is critical to have someone who be an advocate on your behalf. If there are more than one or two physicians involved in your care, have an advocate oversee your use of medications and nutritional supplements. Make sure they are positive, sensible and emotionally supportive. Avoid choosing a worrier, a fretter or someone who is negative. They may inadvertently add more stress to your healing process.

An advocate can be a family member or close friend. It should be someone who you know can help you make clear decisions. He or she should be someone who has stamina and is patient. If you do not have an advocate, and require one, check with the hospital to see if there is an agency that can assist you with your health choices.

BECOMING AN ADVOCATE FOR SOMEONE WHO REQUIRES SURGERY

If a friend or loved one is undergoing surgery and you are the designated advocate, please read this book with an open mind as to the potential benefits of suggested protocols. Even if you are not familiar with acupuncture or other natural medicines, it might be a good time to suspend your judgment and talk to their physician about these natural protocols. If the patient is not permitted to use the nutritional support discussed in this book, you can use the emotional, mental and spiritual support protocols provided. Many patients report very positive results when even a few mind-body protocols are used.

Most importantly, if you are a designated advocate, try to

maintain a positive, caring and cheerful attitude. Encourage the patient to share their emotions and feelings. Being able to express the fear and sadness around the surgery can be liberating. At the same time, it is critical that the advocate not amplify the patient's fears and worries. Instead, direct them to positive and uplifting thoughts, such as a good outcome from the procedure.

Think of yourself as a personal coach. You might want to ask them to focus on something that excites them that they will be able to do when they recover, and keep reminding them. It might be as simple as getting to return home to friends, pets, surroundings. Or it might be a trip they will take or an activity that they can resume. Getting them excited about a future event will be an important focusing mechanism throughout the process of their recovery.

If you are emotionally close to the patient and the surgery is complicated or high risk, you may need your own emotional support during this time. Often advocates put aside their feelings while they are trying to support a patient. It will be important for you to you give yourself extra care and rest, eat well and get counseling if you find yourself feeling overly anxious.

If you are acting as an advocate, you may wish to research the patient's condition by consulting with doctors or through Internet medical sites. Being as informed as possible will assist you in navigating through any decisions that will have to be made throughout the surgical process and the hospital stay.

EMPOWER YOUR HEALING WITH RESEARCH

If you do not require an advocate, research your condition thoroughly if possible or have a friend help you. The Internet provides a wealth of medical sites, trials, studies and reports from trusted sources that can help educate you about your condition.

Avoid websites that make outrageous claims or present short articles that are designed solely to sell you a multitude of products.

Google has a free service called "Google Alerts" that allows you to type in a phrase such as "hip replacement surgery". It will then email you all studies and recent mentions of that subject daily or weekly. The service quickly brings the research to your email inbox.

The more information you gain, the more confidence you will have in making decisions about the scope of your surgery and the alternative protocols that could decrease recovery time and pain. Many of my patients are well informed about their alternatives when they consult with me. Remember, *knowledge is power*. Research offers you more options than you might have realized. These options could make a difference between life and death.

THIS IS YOUR TIME TO NURTURE YOURSELF

This period of preparation prior to surgery may be an important chapter in your life where your commitment to making simple changes such as those outlined in this book will enhance your health, both before and after surgery. I want to empower you to more actively participate in your healing process, both physically and mentally. By making and maintaining changes to your diet, exercise regime and mental outlook, you increase your chances of living a more healthy and balanced life, and possibly avoiding future surgeries and health issues.

Most importantly, you should plan sufficient time to recover, and avoid the temptation to overdo it if your recovery is going well. Consult with your surgeon before engaging in any physical activity or sport.

! TAKE ACTION

After you select your surgeon, download the appropriate questions to ask them at www.recoverquicklyfromsurgery. com/questions

Get a second opinion if the surgery is complicated.

Do necessary research.

If needed, appoint an advocate.

CHAPTER 2

IMPROVING YOUR FITNESS TO ENHANCE RECOVERY

Everyone thinks of changing the world,
but no one thinks of changing himself.

—Leo Tolstoy

Sometimes, the need for surgery arises suddenly. Frequently, however, a patient has weeks or months to prepare. If you have even two weeks before your surgery and are able to exercise, you can increase your fitness level to speed up your recovery time, subject to your physician's approval, of course.

Research shows that getting in better physical shape before your surgery can reduce your need for inpatient rehab significantly. The medical community calls this pre-surgical fitness regime *"prehabilitation"* or "pre-hab" for short. Ideally an exercise program is begun six weeks or more before surgery but a program can be started with less time available, subject to your physician's approval.

Some of the benefits of getting fit before you have surgery include increased circulation and metabolism, faster recovery after surgery, as well as increased general vitality that will carry over into your recovery process. In addition, working out helps rid the body of toxins and metabolic wastes. While you are recovering, your body will expend its energy to heal, rather than trying to detoxify.

Doing some form of exercise also increases serotonin levels, decreases anxiety and releases stress. If you enjoy your workouts you will be more motivated to recover so you can get back to exercise. Patients who have low fitness levels will quickly decline in overall physical health after surgery. Patients with a fit body will take much longer for their fitness levels to decline.

Studies have determined that the typical decline in physical activity that accompanies many surgeries or hospital care causes significant stress to the body and a potential loss of muscle and cardio function following surgery. Because of this, many physicians are recommending pre-hab before surgery—if it is appropriate for the patient.[3] "Pre-hab makes a huge difference in our patients' outcomes," says orthopedic surgeon Hal Crane, MD, founding medical director of the Rose Institute for Joint Replacement at the Rose Medical Center in Denver. "They get vertical sooner and recover faster."

STUDY: Another recent study determined that hip replacement surgery patients who had participated in water- and land-based strength training and aerobic and flexibility exercises for just six weeks prior to their surgeries reduced their odds of needing inpatient rehabilitation by 73 percent.[4]

RECOVERY STARTS BEFORE SURGERY WITH PREHABILITATION

In a 2010 study involving knee surgery, results indicate that the pre-habilitation intervention had a favorable impact on improving functional ability up to 30 percent, increasing knee strength by 50 percent and decreasing pain prior to the left knee operation. Also, prehabilitation increased functional ability and strength prior to surgery and gains in strength were maintained in the non-surgical knee after surgery.[5]

My personal experience supports this research. At the time I underwent surgery, I was very fit from biking, tennis and power yoga which afforded me cardio fitness, good circulation, flexibility and, most importantly, core strength. This expedited my return to physical activity following abdominal surgery and I experienced no loss of function after the five days of recovery.

Orthopedic surgeons maintain that the rewards of pre-habilitation are evident in the first 24 hours following surgery. "Even in a fairly brief time period, the exercise paid off for the participants," says Daniel Rooks, Ph.D., Assistant Professor of Medicine at Harvard Medical School. "Their level of function and pain stabilized prior to surgery, whereas those who did not exercise got worse. The benefits of exercise before surgery are very clear: the more you can do for yourself physically before surgery, the better off you will be."[6]

Consult with your surgeon to determine if there are any health concerns with engaging in mild to moderate exercise prior to your surgery. Overdoing exercise before a procedure might present a risk to certain conditions, so it is best to get clearance from your surgeon.

HOW MUCH AND WHAT KIND OF EXERCISE IS OPTIMUM?

The nature and frequency of exercise will depend on your overall level of health and fitness as well as the issue for which you require surgery. If exercise is appropriate for you, your physician and natural health care practitioner can help create an exercise plan for you. If you are having knee surgery, for example, you may be able to swim or work out at the gym without risking further injury to your knee.

THE THREE TYPES OF FITNESS THAT CAN HELP YOU RECOVER FASTER

The three ways to enhance your fitness level include *cardiovascular fitness*, *strength training*, and *flexibility training* such as yoga and stretching. It is ideal to utilize all three forms to be truly fit. Most professional athletes use cross-training exercises in all forms of fitness. Your surgeon will advise you about appropriate limitations. Even if you engage in short walks or simple stretching, you can enhance the outcome of your procedure.

As we review these three types of fitness, begin planning what you can do to increase your post-operative results.

CARDIOVASCULAR FITNESS

Cardiovascular activities increase blood flow throughout the body, drain lymphatic congestion, increase heart strength and reduce tension. If your condition is not heart-related or restricted by a muscular-skeletal issue, ask your surgeon if you may walk or swim for exercise.

I usually recommend that people find a form of exercise that they enjoy and that can be done on a regular basis. Health permitting, engaging in a variety of workouts keeps you interested and avoids injuries from overuse in one area.

Walking

If you are able, walking may be the simplest way to increase your cardiovascular fitness. You may make walking more interesting by listening to motivating music as well as walking in beautiful and interesting areas.

If you are currently not fit, start slowly and begin walking a comfortable distance, increasing it daily. In even a short time, you will see a change in your general fitness and well-being.

There are several ways to remain motivated to engage in a pre-hab fitness regime. Follow any or all of these suggestions to immediately begin preparing to recover quickly.

1. **Increase your walking distance with a mental rehearsal of your route.** After engaging in a walk, sit or lie down and visualize walking the entire route again in as much detail as possible. Imagine yourself enjoying it. The next time you walk, your subconscious will believe it already has walked double the distance. You will easily want to walk a few more blocks. This

visualization technique helps you to increase your endurance.

Research indicates that both physical and psychological reactions in certain situations can be improved with visualization. Such repeated imagery can build both experience and confidence, especially for an athlete's ability to perform certain skills under competitive circumstances. For example, a professional athlete might mentally rehearse or "run" the entire race in a visualization technique in their mind the night before the actual race. You can do the same with walking or any form of exercise to increase the endurance in your mind first.[7]

2. **Purchase an inexpensive stopwatch.** Time your walks and decide to decrease the amount of time it takes to do your walk. As this happens, you will then have time to increase the length of your walks. Increase the distance or speed until you are walking a minimum of thirty minutes at a fast clip. Even as you "get up to speed", you can try to take seconds off. It is very rewarding to see that you are improving daily.

3. **Walk in an area that has more hills.** The greater the incline, the more you build cardio-fitness. If you live in an area with hiking trails, consider hiking as a means to fitness that will provide you with a dose of serenity.

4. **Establish a realistic goal.** When you decide to start a walking or exercise program, pick a goal that challenges you but is not beyond your reach. Your surgeon will guide you in restrictions.

5. **Indoor Cardio.** In areas where inclement weather prevails, there are gyms that offer treadmills and cross-training cardio equipment. If these are new to you, ask a fitness trainer for advice.

Other Forms of Cardio Fitness

Some people are prohibited from walking and may enjoy swimming.

Swimming can be very relaxing as well as a great fitness builder. Utilize a variety of strokes to increase your fitness. If you are not a strong swimmer, you can hold onto a kickboard.

Water aerobics workouts are geared for those who need to increase their fitness levels gradually. The buoyancy and resistance offered by the water allows for strengthening yet gentle conditioning.

Other cardiovascular exercise options include biking, rowing, dancing and fitness or aerobics classes.

Be sure to consult your surgeon and other physicians if you have any doubts about engaging in a fitness program. Some people will not be well enough to engage in exercise. But even if you are only able to take short walks, implementing a plan to walk a few blocks a couple of times per week, in most cases will help with the post-surgery recovery time.

STRENGTH TRAINING

In the weeks prior to surgery, strength or resistance training, such as lifting weights, may be extremely beneficial to your recovery time. Most gyms employ a fitness trainer who is very knowledgeable about strengthening exercises. Consult with your physician or healthcare practitioner about any restrictions in strength training.

You can use dumbbells, pulleys, band resistance straps or weight machines at your gym. If you are over fifty-five years of age, you may want to use weight machines instead of free weights or barbells as they offer more stability and even weight distribution, which will help in preventing injuries. Combining weight training with aerobic exercise is a winning combination for improved fitness.

A regular regime of strength training can increase bone density and decrease the risk of bone fractures in older patients. It may increase overall strength, energy level and endurance as well as help burn calories more efficiently. In addition, studies suggest that it can reduce surgical pain and might reduce the potential for developing for blood clots.[8]

Depending on your health issue, age and level of fitness, the amount of weights and frequency or repetitions will vary. Prior to leg surgery, for example, you might want to strengthen your abdominal muscles and upper body with some attention to your legs, if your physician approves. A certified athletic trainer should be able to design a custom exercise program with your surgery in mind.

If your doctor deems it appropriate, I suggest doing abdominal strengthening exercises to build your core strength. This may be especially important to those who are having abdominal surgery. Toned muscles will have a better blood supply and will heal more rapidly after surgery. It will be much more difficult to strengthen them after surgery if there are any major incisions.

FLEXIBILITY TRAINING

The third form of essential exercise is flexibility training. Stretching, Pilates and yoga are several forms of strength and flexibility training.

Yoga is currently very popular in the U.S. Standing, sitting or reclining postures are performed individually or they may flow one into the other. Breathing is a very important aspect of yoga and is used by practitioners to perform the postures. What makes yoga so popular among people of all ages?

- It strengthens, relaxes, and tones the muscles.

- It increases flexibility.

- It strengthens the *vital force,* allowing us to heal more quickly.

- It increases blood flow to internal organs and glands.

- It reduces stress and relaxes both body and mind.

Studies show that yoga increases mental acuity. After nine months of yoga, developmentally challenged children showed improvement in general mental ability, psychomotor coordination and intelligence and social behavior.[9]

Yoga also can reduce pain in your body and add years to your life. A recent 2011 study documented more than 100 people with low back pain. One group attended a weekly yoga class, the second focused on aerobic and strengthening exercises, and the third read a self-care book on back pain. After 12 weeks, patients in the yoga group reported better back function. At 26 weeks, they also reported less pain.[10]

Lastly, some research indicates yoga can decrease depression, stress and anxiety. Researchers at the University of Utah noted that people who have a poorly regulated response to stress are also more sensitive to pain. The study concluded that yoga, as one technique, can help a person regulate their stress and, therefore, pain responses.[11] Most importantly, yoga can provide a spiritual deepening and a sense of peace, relaxation and renewal during a stressful time in your life. Yoga may not be appropriate for everyone or for your condition, so get your physician's approval first.

Athletic trainers will teach a variety of exercises and stretches to help their clients maximize fitness. Pilates is another form of stretching and strengthening using specific floor exercises and machines. It usually requires an instructor.

Energetic Fitness

For centuries, Eastern traditions have taught series of postures, movements and exercises that increase flexibility and promote inner vitality and tranquility while balancing the nervous system. Many of the movements are not physically strenuous and offer a different kind of fitness from the other forms discussed. Generally, the ancient arts of Tai Chi (pronounced "tie-chee") and Qi Gong (pronounced "chee-gong") are done standing and involve performing a series of gentle, precise and fluid movements. These movements have the ability to focus your energy, create internal and physical balance as well as promote well-being. Research shows that Tai Chi can reduce pain and improve physical function, self-efficiency, depression, and the health-related quality of life for knee osteoarthritis.[12]

Multiple research studies indicate the tremendous health benefits of Tai Chi and Qi Gong. These practices may be done by yourself or in a group. You may find a practicing group locally and try a few sessions with an experienced instructor. In preparing for surgery, these exercises will help you feel more relaxed, calm and may help you sleep more deeply.

! TAKE ACTION

Ask your surgeon if you are able to increase your fitness level.

Walk, swim or engage in cardio if your condition allows.

Do some light yoga or athletic stretching.

CHANGE YOUR LIFESTYLE AND RECOVER QUICKLY

Change before you have to.

—Jack Welch

RESEARCH REVEALS THE SECRETS TO HEALING FASTER

If your surgery is not emergent and you have time to prepare, now would be an excellent time to quit smoking. You may not have realized how smoking can negatively affect your outcome and recovery. If your medical doctor has not already stressed the importance of this critical change, perhaps this book will inspire you to use this surgical "opportunity" as an impetus to stop smoking.

Research indicates that the effects of smoking are one of the strongest deterrents to healing quickly.[13] The most significant factor for shortening your recovery time as well as reducing pain and swelling can depend on the amount of inflammation in your body. Tobacco residues promote inflammation in the body. Furthermore, smoking stresses the lungs, liver, heart and the lymphatic system, all of which need to be in optimum functioning order to heal properly and quickly. It is especially important to quit smoking before having a surgery that could be life threatening.

STUDY: UT Southwestern Medical Center reports a study that establishes that people who smoke regularly have a higher percentage of surgical complications and do not heal as quickly. Dr. Rod Rohrich, University of Texas Southwestern's chairman of plastic surgery, says that smoking not only reduces the body's capacity for wound healing, it also raises the risk for complications after surgery.[14]

WHY SMOKING IMPAIRS RECOVERY

The chemicals in tobacco smoke interfere with the filtering mechanism in the lungs, causing less oxygen in the blood. Smoking also reduces blood flow. That means there's less oxygen-rich blood flowing to tissues throughout the body. Blood flow and oxygen are essential for the healing process, and without that oxygen-rich blood, you won't heal as well or as quickly.

STUDY: A recent 2010 Swedish medical study analyzed the effects of smoking before surgery, concluding that a smoking cessation intervention program during the first six weeks after acute fracture surgery decreases the risk of postoperative complications by nearly half.[15]

Other reports state that patients who smoke in the 24 hours before their surgery have a dangerous decrease in blood oxygen levels during surgery. This could prevent major organs from getting the necessary supply of oxygen. Smoking reduces oxygen supply to organs because of chemical reactions that take place when the carbon monoxide from smoke gets into the bloodstream. This carbon monoxide effect is temporary, so smokers who abstain from cigarettes in the 24 hours before surgery have the same risk of low oxygen supply to the heart as nonsmokers.

Physicians should warn patients not to smoke before surgery in the same way they warn patients to not eat. If smokers are not warned, they may be even more likely to smoke since they cannot eat before surgery.

Even using the patch is problematic, unless you are using it to quit. The patch will deliver nicotine to your body, which in turn will impair healing.

WHAT MAKES SMOKING SO HARMFUL?

Tobacco smoke contains many harmful chemicals including ammonia, arsenic, benzene formaldehyde and hydrogen cyanide. In addition, tar, nicotine and carbon monoxide are all found in smoke and are linked with causing disease.

- Tar contains ingredients known to cause cancer in animals. Close to 70 percent of the tar contained in cigarette smoke is deposited in the lungs.

- Nicotine can constrict blood vessels, increase blood pressure and heart rate and can change overall blood composition and metabolism.

- Carbon monoxide is a lethal gas found in cigarette smoke. By combining with hemoglobin (the oxygen-carrying substance in blood) it becomes particularly dangerous in combination with surgery. Carbon monoxide can also negatively affect the electrical activity of the heart.

Many medical practitioners have observed that smokers take longer to heal, and some surgeons will not operate on those who continue to smoke. Typically, smokers are more prone to inflammation in and around joint areas, which will cause an increase in pain.

Hypnosis, acupuncture and positive affirmations have been used to help people stop smoking. I personally know people who, after smoking for sixty years, were able to stop "cold turkey". So can you.

PASSIVE SMOKING

If you are around someone who smokes and thereby are exposed to

43

passive smoke, remove yourself from this environment. Side stream smoke comes from the burning end of the cigarette and is not filtered. The U.S. Environmental Protection Agency has declared passive smoking or exposure to environmental tobacco smoke (ETS) to be a "Class A Carcinogen" which means that it is capable of causing cancer in humans. The 2006 U.S. Surgeon General's report states that secondhand smoke causes premature death and disease in children and in adults who do not smoke.[16]

If you live with a smoker, ask them to smoke outside, as your life could depend on it.

ARE YOU READY TO QUIT SMOKING?

Because it can be extremely difficult to quit smoking, I recommend getting professional assistance to support you. Making the commitment to quit smoking is a landmark life decision—it is important to ask for help during this difficult undertaking.

As an important resource, visit www.smokefree.gov. It offers a variety of information, including live experts, to guide you. You should seek out local support groups and programs and talk to your physician so that you will have a solid plan to quit and remain free from your smoking habit.

For alternative support, you may find a local acupuncturist or naturopathic doctor who can provide a stop-smoking protocol that helps with cravings and anxiety through the use of natural herbs and supplements. Hypnotherapy has proven helpful for some. If you have enough time before surgery, you can use the nicotine patch. Just remember, the patch should not be used in the month before surgery.

I recall a woman who used affirmations to quit smoking. Every day that she lit up a cigarette for the eight weeks leading up to her birthday she proclaimed, "On or before my birthday, I am a non-smoker". She succeeded in quitting before her birthday. I have shared this with various patients and many have used this approach successfully.

CAFFEINE AND RAPID RECOVERY

Caffeine comes in many forms. In addition to coffee and tea, it is added to sodas, carbonated drinks and energy drinks. Green tea is said to have between 15-40 milligrams of caffeine and black tea averages about 50 milligrams per eight ounce cup.[17] Chocolate contains a small amount of caffeine. It may also be found in some over-the-counter medications such as Anacin, Excedrin and Motrin.

Caffeine breaks down capillary walls and encourages bleeding. As enjoyable as it may be, it taxes your liver and can cause hypertension and other issues later in life. Thus, one should not consume caffeine before your operation. Don't feel badly if you are addicted, as you are not alone: approximately 80 percent of Americans use caffeine.

Quitting suddenly before an operation could give you a strong headache. I recommend quitting caffeine one or two weeks prior to surgery. To prevent headaches, wean off of caffeine by drinking about one quarter less of your caffeine intake per day over a five to seven day period, two weeks before your surgery. Switch to non-caffeinated hot drinks such as hot water and lemon or drink herbal, non-caffeinated tea. I recommend Teechino and Caffix as coffee substitutes because they are gluten free.

You should ideally allow two weeks to give yourself time to acclimate to your new caffeine-free diet. Without caffeine, you will sleep more deeply and find a new way to enjoy your life without the addiction to an artificial stimulant. If you are having a tough time getting up, you may have adrenal insufficiency. Talk to your holistic health care provider for advice on what supplements to take to boost your adrenal system.

If you are unable to function without caffeine, limit your consumption of coffee to less than one cup per day or drink green tea, which has a milder form of caffeine and has documented health benefits.

ALCOHOL AND YOUR RECOVERY

Since alcohol causes dehydration as well as stressing the liver and other organs, it is ideal to refrain from drinking alcohol for one to two weeks before surgery.

Alcohol is an inflammatory agent. If recovering quickly and with less pain is your intention, note the study below. Remember, your liver has to work overtime to remove the alcohol from your blood stream. After years of working overtime, it begins to store the toxins from alcohol in fat cells. This leads to a fatty liver, which in time, will lead to cirrhosis of the liver, a deadly disease.

Your liver will need to be functioning at a high level to detoxify the anesthetic and other drugs that you will need to take after your surgery. Giving your liver a rest from daily alcohol use will enable it to function at a higher level when you will most need it.

STUDY: A recent clinical study proved the negative effects of alcohol on surgery patients. Claudia Spies, an intensive care specialist at the Charité University hospital in Berlin, said: "A significantly high rate of complications can develop in patients who consume alcohol at levels that are less than excessive." She further stated that about "20 percent of adults admitted to hospital drink three beers or two glasses of wine every day for a prolonged period, and they were more likely to fall victim to pneumonia or heart muscle disease or suffer complications such as bleeding after surgery." "In addition," Spies said, "some 50 percent of patients who are committed to hospitals after an accident suffered their injuries under the influence of alcohol. Consequently, the rate of immune-system complications in emergency medicine is also very high."[18]

The article also cites Elizabeth Kovacs, director of the alcohol research program at Loyola University Medical Center in Illinois who says: "More alcohol abusers die of pulmonary infections than liver cirrhosis." The article further mentions an important study that proves that mice exposed to alcohol and pneumonia bacteria could not fight off the pneumonia as well as a group of mice that were exposed only to the pneumonia and not the alcohol. Since drinking can weaken the immunities, you may want to eliminate all alcohol in advance of your surgery.

! TAKE ACTION

Stop smoking.

Reduce caffeine.

Reduce or eliminate alcohol before your surgery.

HEAL FASTER WITH THE RECOVER QUICKLY DIET

Life expectancy would grow by leaps and bounds if green vegetables smelled as good as bacon

—Doug Larson

Your pre-surgery goal should be to reduce as much inflammation as possible in your system before and after your procedure. An anti-inflammatory diet is your first step to reducing the amount of swelling caused by surgery. Less swelling will result in less pain, a shortened recovery time and a lowered risk of post-surgical complications. Just ask a cosmetic surgeon how inflammation negatively impacts the result of their cosmetic surgery.

WHY THIS SPECIFIC DIET CAN ENHANCE YOUR RECOVERY

Inflammation is now recognized as the underlying cause of most chronic diseases, including heart disease, arthritis, cancer and autoimmune diseases.

COMMON SYMPTOMS OF INFLAMMATION

Wrinkles	Arthritis
Infections	Knee Pain
Acid Reflux	Joint Pain
Cancer	Back Pain
Psoriasis	Headaches
Acne	Scarring

49

Chronic inflammation also lowers the effectiveness of the immune system to fight all forms of infections. Most people will die from a chronic disease or an infection.

Diseases linked to chronic inflammation include: Alzheimer's, attention deficit disorder, autism, chronic allergies, anemia, various forms of cancer, Crohn's disease, migraines and other headache syndromes, skin disorders, epilepsy, weakened immune system, thyroid issues, irritable bowel syndrome (IBS), autoimmune disorders such as lupus, chronic fatigue syndrome and rheumatoid arthritis, and even mental disorders such as schizophrenia and chronic depression.

In addition, inflammation increases pain. The longer you are in pain after a surgical procedure, the longer your recovery time. Reduce your inflammation and swelling, and you should shorten your recovery time. In addition, ongoing inflammation can increase the need for painkillers or anti-inflammatory medications which can have negative side effects.

THE MAIN CAUSES OF INFLAMMATION

Inflammation is your body's response to stress. Environmental factors, such as allergens, heavy metals, pesticides, as well as airborne and waterborne toxins, stress the body as they accumulate, creating inflammation in the joints and organs. Dietary stressors such sugar, gluten, processed foods, red meat, junk food, caffeine products, sodas and alcohol can also create inflammation in the body.

External stressors that create inflammation include lack of sleep, dehydration and overdoing physical activity. Work, family and financial issues act as emotional stressors. Any or all of these stresses can be accumulative taking their toll on the body's ability to recover quickly.

Therefore it is extremely important to moderate any stresses that we can control. Eating a healthy, non-inflammatory diet is the primary way inflammation can be controlled, just as it is important to reduce as much life stress as possible. The Recover Quickly Diet is specifically designed to shorten your recovery time and reduce pain levels.

WHY AN ANTI-INFLAMMATORY DIET ACCELERATES RECOVERY

The typical modern diet is comprised of an excessive amount of sugar, processed foods, unhealthy fats, starchy carbohydrates, alcohol, preservatives and pesticides. These dietary factors collectively lead to systemic inflammation and toxicity. This inflammation will increase the amount of pain you will experience after your surgery.

Most Western cultures have migrated away from simpler fare of farm-grown meat and vegetables. Our supermarkets are filled with an array of packaged foods that are replete with sugary, starchy, fatty or processed ingredients. Preservatives, artificial sweeteners and pesticide levels are not well-regulated.

Most Europeans and Americans consume up to 90 percent acidifying foods such as meat, dairy, sugars, grains and starches. When the body pH is acidic, it is more prone to inflammation. The body's chemistry seeks homeostasis, and all systems are geared to keeping the blood at the perfect pH of 7.1. Anything less than that is acidic, anything more is alkaline. When the diet consists mostly of acidic foods, the body has to work very hard to maintain proper pH levels. This puts a strain on the body, which in turn encumbers the recovery process after surgery or illness.

Even foods that are considered "healthy" can cause inflammation in the body. Health foods can be over processed and contain soy, wheat, dairy and other foods that may cause inflammation.

Caffeine and alcohol consumption, even in moderate amounts, stress the body. In addition, sugar and other ingredients are added to these beverages. Sodas are particularly inflammatory, full of empty calories with no nutritional value.

With such a plethora of food and beverage choices, it can be difficult to make the appropriate choices that will accelerate recovery from surgery.

This chapter offers dietary guidelines that will guide you in limiting your intake of inflammatory foods as well as promoting foods and other nutrients that will nourish important functions of the body. Ideally, you will make this your diet for life. If you choose to do so, you will feel energized and more balanced. In addition, the Recovery Quickly Diet will lower your risk of developing a chronic disease or infection, as well as the need for further surgery.

The health food industry has developed many foods that are a delicious alternative to processed, pesticide-filled, overly sweet and preservative tainted foods. Your best choices will always be fresh, organic, unprocessed foods that are raw or cooked to perfection.

I suggest following this diet for two to four weeks before your surgery and as many weeks after your procedure that it takes to recover. Every change you make in your diet is a step towards recovering quickly from surgery.

STUDY: Oncologists report that cancer patients with the lowest amounts of inflammation were twice as likely as the other patients to live through the next several years.[19]

THE RECOVER QUICKLY DIET

1. **Consume fresh, organic vegetables as 50–75 percent of your meals.** Vegetables contain fiber, vitamins, minerals and enzymes in high density, and are generally well assimilated by the body. In addition, vegetables alkalinize the blood and thereby reduce inflammation. Choose brightly-colored organic vegetables that are fresh. Include raw salads at least once a day. In order to retain the nutrients, do not overcook your vegetables.

2. **Eat fresh fruits as snacks.** Fruits serve as healthy snacks containing fiber as well as essential vitamins. Berries, grapefruit, greener bananas, pears and apples are optimum because they have a lower glycemic index. It is best to consume them before a meal or between meals as they digest more rapidly than protein and may cause fermentation in the digestive tract.

3. **Eat organically raised poultry, eggs and wild-caught fish.** The body requires the proper amino acids to heal. These are best found in organic lean protein. Low quality, processed, cured and fatty meats may contain harmful hormones, additives, preservatives and pesticides that can inhibit your body's recovery process. Eat a variety of proteins so that you get a balance of amino acids. Those with kidney issues need to discuss the appropriate protein intake with their doctor.

   DOES ORGANIC REALLY MATTER?

   A recent study showed that workers in French wine vineyards who were regularly exposed to pesticides in the grapes had an increased risk of brain tumors.[20]

4. **Limit red meat.** Red meat is high in fat, usually contains hormones and is rarely organically fed. Additionally, red meat is

high in Omega 6's and low in Omega 3's, which may contribute to inflammation.

Animals raised as a food source are often treated with hormones like estradiol and zeranol in order to fatten them. These growth enhancers are known endocrine disruptors and have been shown to enhance human breast tumor cells.[21]

5. **Minimize starches such as potatoes, rice and beans.** Starches add extra calories and not enough nutrients, unless you are very active or a vegetarian. Proper combinations of rice and beans may contain enough protein if you are a vegan.

6. **Avoid gluten products.** During the last 20 years, the wheat kernel has been genetically modified to contain more protein. Unfortunately, this made the gluten within the wheat grain less digestible. This has caused certain people with specific genetic serotypes to be gluten intolerant. Unfortunately, 60 percent of all Americans may be intolerant of the gluten molecule, causing inflammatory diseases to express themselves as they age. Specifically, it is thought that those with blood type O may be more intolerant to both gluten, causing inflammation in the small intestines, which then disrupt proper assimilation of nutrients.

Gluten is found in whole wheat, white bread flour, rye, barley and spelt, and acts as an inflammatory agent for many people. While some people have undetected gluten intolerance, others may be affected with joint swelling, bloating, sneezing, itchy eyes, loose bowels, stomach pain, flatulence, achy joints, back pain, blood sugar imbalances and more. Continued use of gluten products for these patients can later cause celiac disease, a chronic condition of the small intestines, which occurs in one in 133 individuals.

Also, more commonly, people can experience an immune reaction to gliadin, which is contained in gluten products. This sensitivity causes the improper digestion of gluten. Your immune system, believing it to be hostile, attacks the gliadin, leaving large holes in your digestive track. This results in inflammation and a breakdown of the immune system. This inflammation can affect your joints, gut and the area around your incisions.

> " Many of my patients, that have removed gluten and wheat from their diet have noticed their joint pains disappear in a week."

Products such as baked goods, pastas, snack foods, gravies, pastries and many processed foods contain wheat products that contain gluten. Read labels before purchasing. Substitute amaranth, buckwheat, corn, millet, quinoa and brown or wild rice. There are increasingly more gluten free products available as people are recognizing the effects of gluten on their health.

7. **Avoid sugar in all forms.** Sugar acts as a major contributor of inflammation in the body. If you want to reduce inflammation and increase your energy overall, you must reduce sugar intake. A recent 2009 study linked high insulin levels (thereby high sugar levels) with increased risk of breast cancer. In this report, women who had higher insulin levels had nearly twice the risk of developing breast cancer as women with the lowest insulin levels.[22] Numerous other studies have linked high glucose sugar levels with the promotion of cancer cells.

In addition, sugar may cause loss of tissue elasticity, which is important in healing after surgery. It interferes with the absorption of calcium and magnesium, leads to chromium deficiency and upsets the relationship of other minerals in the body.

High blood sugar is linked to heart disease and diabetes. Both of these present a risk to anyone having surgery. It is also linked to health issues such as a suppressed immune system, hyperactivity, depression, mineral deficiencies, acidity, obesity, arthritis, gum and tooth disease, food allergies, fluid retention and headaches.[23]

High fructose corn syrup, refined sugar and foods that have a high glycemic index should be avoided. Drinks with sugar or artificial sweeteners and caffeine offer no nutrition, supply empty calories, are inflammatory and dehydrate the body.

AVOID SUGARY BEVERAGES

Beverages such as sodas containing sugar and caffeine, sugared ice teas, coffee drinks and juices with added sugar, do not satisfy the body's need for water to properly hydrate. They introduce large amounts of sugar into the blood stream quickly. If they contain caffeine, they may also act as diuretics, causing dehydration as well as a spike in blood sugar.

Your body needs water to function properly. It needs two quarts per day, best consumed between meals. Hydrate with pure water, not tap water. Add lemon to pure water for a refreshing beverage.

Need a lift? Brew some green tea, add a few tablespoons each of pomegranate and blueberry juice, chill and sip it during the day. Try adding small amounts of stevia or acacia honey (a type of honey that has lower glycemic levels) to your foods if you want them sweeter.

Examples of food or beverages to be avoided include candy, cakes, pastries, ice cream, sodas, white rice, white flour, alcohol and sweetened beverages.

8. **Minimize dairy, especially those from cow.** There are many reasons why it is important to avoid or limit dairy, especially as an adult. Increasingly, dairy is linked to an increased cancer risk due to the 50 plus hormones that occur naturally or are artificially introduced into the cow. Dairy products introduce high levels of cholesterol into the body leading to cardiovascular issues. Various populations in the U.S. have an allergy or intolerance to cow dairy products leading to digestive issues. Because dairy molecules are not easily broken down in the gut, consumption may cause mucus formation in the body.

The calcium in milk products doesn't necessarily build bone mass. The protein in milk competes with the calcium for absorption into bone. There are much better sources of calcium in eggshells and vegetables. The phosphorus in milk products ages cell structure. In addition, there are likely to be a variety of contaminants such as pesticides, herbicides, antibiotic residues and other drugs used to treat the cows.

Dairy also contains Omega 6 fats, an essential fatty acid. However, the American diet is higher in Omega 6 than Omega 3 EFAs. An imbalance in this ratio is known to produce chronic inflammation.

Goat and sheep dairy molecules are smaller, thereby easier to digest properly. Use small amounts of goat and sheep cheese as a condiment. Instead of milk, try drinking rice milk, coconut milk or almond milk. If you enjoy the taste of butter, try making ghee or clarified butter as this process removes the dairy solids.

SUBSTITUTES FOR DAIRY

Goat dairy (try to find local)
Sheep's milk cheese (feta, Manchego)
Almond milk (organic, unsweetened best)
Rice dream (organic)
Cashew milk (make your own)
Coconut milk (good for cooking)
Raw unpasteurized cow's milk (whole foods)
Nut milks made in a vita-mix or blender
Ghee (butter with milk solids removed-make your own)

9. Avoid processed, junk and fast foods. Processed and junk foods such as chips, breakfast cereals, frozen dinners, cookies, pastries and crackers are usually made with wheat, sugars, preservatives, soy bean or cottonseed oil, MSG, excessive sodium and other unhealthy ingredients.

Most fast foods contain high levels of fat and sodium, including trans fats, which are known to be carcinogenic. They are usually high in calories, non-organic and may be deep fried in fats that are rancid.

BOTTOM LINE: *These foods do not offer real nutrition and readily cause inflammation in the body. Avoid before surgery.*

---

10. **Avoid foods with high sodium content.** Excessive sodium will cause swelling, high blood pressure, hypertension and fluid retention. If you are able to minimize swelling during your procedure, you will minimize pain. Most labels list sodium content and state the percentage of the recommended daily limit for sodium consumption.

11. **Avoid consuming foods from the nightshade family.** A recent study indicates that consuming nightshade vegetables (potatoes,

tomatoes, eggplant, paprika, peppers, tomatillos, pimentos, tobacco sauce, ground cherries, etc) may delay the healing process after surgery. It is suggested that the nightshade vegetables inhibit two important enzymes that process the anesthesia drugs. Nightshades also contain solanine, which is said to be toxic and may increase joint pain, and alkaloids, which may compromise joint function.[24] Although the nightshade vegetables may not adversely affect everyone, it might be wise to avoid or limit your consumption of them prior to your surgery.

12. Avoid or limit fish with high mercury content. Mercury and other heavy metals are inflammatory and may cause cancer and other degenerative diseases. Albacore tuna, swordfish and shark are the most common fish that retain mercury in their flesh. Lower mercury levels are found in salmon, scallops, mackerel, lighter fleshed tuna, shrimp, shellfish and catfish.[25]

13. Eat plenty of fruits and vegetables to alkalinize your system. An acidic imbalance can lessen the body's ability to absorb minerals and other necessary nutrients, as well as decrease its ability to repair damaged cells. It also decreases its ability to detoxify heavy metals, which makes it more susceptible to inflammation.

Specific vegetables should be eaten or juiced regularly to aid in reducing inflammation. Dark, leafy greens, collards, parsley, alfalfa, bean sprouts and celery are known to be key vegetables that restore a proper alkaline balance. Studies show that juicing celery can prevent high blood pressure, prevent gout and help arthritis. Celery contains more than a dozen anti-inflammatory agents, including apigenin, a COX 2-inhibiting compound similar to some anti-inflammatory drugs. Juicing it will optimize its effects.[26]

14. Consume several small meals a day. Eating several small meals that contain 15 to 20 grams of light protein will help maintain the proper blood sugar levels, providing steady energy throughout the day. It is optimum also to consume 20 grams of vegetables with each meal. Include healthy oils, such as olive, flax and coconut, as well as other essential fatty acids found in fish oil.

15. Enjoy healthy fats. It is best to cook with olive oil, canola oil or coconut oil. Healthy fats are necessary for hormone production yet may add a high caloric factor to foods. Examples of good fats are cold-water fish, walnut, olive, canola and coconut oil, seeds, nuts and avocados.

It is also important to supplement Omega 3 if you are not eating salmon and other cold-water fish.

16. Avoid soy products especially soy protein. The health food industry, seeking to provide a vegetarian protein, discovered ways to process soybeans to produce soy protein isolate, a product that can be used to make protein bars and other health foods. Many nutritionists do not consider this a healthy, digestible food. The soybean must be processed with extreme heat and chemicals to produce soymilk and cheese. Tofu and other soy products such as soymilk can act like estrogen and may cause problems for both men and women.

Soy sauce contains wheat and therefore gluten, as well as an increased amount of sodium. Tamari, a fermented soy sauce is gluten free with less sodium, is fine to use as a condiment.

17. Enjoy these anti-inflammatory herbs. Research shows that the following herbs reduce inflammation in the body.

Green tea is a delicious way to begin the day. Numerous clinical studies show that the ingredient in green tea, ECGC can block chemical pathways that can lead to cancer cell growth. More research indicates that green tea extract also acts as a powerful antioxidant and anti-inflammatory, and has been shown to help control leukemia.[27] Taking green tea in a liquid extract form in a smoothie or drinking several cups of green tea daily may help prevent inflammation and act as a powerful antioxidant.

Turmeric is part of the ginger family and a main spice in yellow curry dishes. It is known to be one of the most effective anti-inflammatory food ingredients. It contains a molecule known as curcumin, which studies have shown to inhibit cancer growth.[28] Dissolve in olive oil, mix with black pepper and add to rice, salad dressing or curry dishes. Try adding to a smoothie in the morning. You can buy it in capsule form as well.

Ginger acts as both an anti-inflammatory and antioxidant. It can thin your blood so it is best to consult with your physician before using it right before your surgery. Ginger tea helps digestion after a meal. Grate and add to your vegetables, soups, juice or tea.

THE RECOVER QUICKLY DIET IN REVIEW

- Consume fresh, organic vegetables as 50 to 75 percent of your meals.

- Eat fresh fruits as snacks.

- Eat organically raised poultry, eggs and wild-caught fish.

- Limit red meat.

- Moderate consumption of potatoes, rice and beans.

- Avoid gluten (wheat) products.

- Avoid sugar in all forms.

- Minimize dairy, especially cow dairy products.

- Avoid processed, junk and fast foods.

- Avoid foods with high sodium content.

- Avoid consuming foods from the nightshade family.

- Avoid or limit fish with high mercury content.

- Eat several small meals a day.

- Use anti-inflammatory herbs such as green tea, turmeric, ginger.

As an added benefit, eating the Recover Quickly Diet may help you lose weight.

❗ TAKE ACTION

Eliminate gluten, sugar and dairy.

Eat healthy protein and organic vegetables two to three meals a day.

Remove junk food from your diet for two or more weeks before surgery.

CHAPTER 5

THE ESSENTIAL TWO DRINKS TO ACCELERATE RECOVERY

If I'd known I was going to live so long,
I'd have taken better care of myself

—Leon Eldred

WATER: THE FOUNTAIN OF RECOVERY

Our bodies are comprised predominately of water. A well-hydrated body will heal faster. The most important advice that I can give to anyone having surgery is make sure that you are well hydrated in the weeks before and after surgery, especially the day before, as you may not be allowed to drink water twelve hours before any major surgery.

Water has a multitude of powerful effects on our bodies. It can be a neutral medium that acts to hydrate the body and is a key ingredient to optimum health. Although the average body mass is 57 percent water on the average, it can be as low as 45 percent in aged and obese people. The need for continual hydration is illustrated by the fact that most humans will survive less than a week without water.

THE POWER OF WATER AS A DETOXIFYING AGENT

Water is one of the first medicinal agents to take once you are in recovery. In addition to your body's normal water requirements, it now has the extra load of detoxifying and eliminating the residue of anesthesia and medications used before, during and after surgery. If you are not allowed to drink water immediately following surgery, sucking on an ice cube will begin the hydration process.

Water can be toxic to the body if it contains viral or bacterial agents, heavy metals and noxious agents such as chlorine, fluoride or chromium 6. Try not to drink unfiltered tap water, especially in cities.

Water can become a detoxifying agent that can serve as a scavenging agent, drawing out heavy metals as well as detoxifying the body. It also serves to purify the body by diluting toxins and assisting in the excretion of bodily wastes.

If you think your system might be toxic from exposure to external pesticides, toxins and medications or from an unhealthy lifestyle that includes excess sugar, alcohol or smoking, you should increase your water intake in the weeks before your surgery.

If your lymphatic system becomes congested as a result of poor eating habits, sipping hot water with lemon juice throughout the day can be very healing to your system. Even drinking hot water by itself can increase your metabolism and allow your body to detox very gently. Please note that lemon water has a different effect on the body and should not replace drinking purified water.

WHEN AND HOW TO HYDRATE TO OPTIMIZE YOUR RECOVERY

In order to expedite your recovery time, your body requires a minimum of a quart of water two times per day in between meals for a week or two. If you weigh more than 200 pounds, you will need to increase that amount.

Water that has anything else in it is not pure water. Therefore, consuming tea, coffee or flavored drinks do not constitute drinking water. In fact, coffee and tea are diuretics, causing excessive elimination of water from your body.

Drinking liquids at meals, even if it is water, is not always beneficial for some people. It can dilute enzymes needed to digest the food that you are eating. I prefer people to drink large amounts of water in-between meals and small amounts with meals.

Also, unless it is a hot day, it is advisable to use little or no ice. Your body attempts to maintain a certain internal body temperature to facilitate metabolism and proper function. Drinking chilled liquids puts an undue stress on the body.

The body will often signal hunger when it is in fact thirsty; therefore, it is a good idea to fill a liter water bottle with purified water and sip throughout the day. Drinking a small amount just before you lay down to sleep can also help hydrate the body while you are sleeping.

If you do indulge in caffeinated and alcoholic drinks, make sure you double your efforts to hydrate. Many people feel the negative effects of alcohol largely due to dehydration. Drink more water if you live in a dry climate or high altitude location.

CHOOSE THE PUREST SOURCES OF WATER

Do not drink tap water, as it can contain too many pollutants, additives and bacteria. Drink water that is distilled or run through a reverse osmosis or other filter. Distilled water does not contain the viruses, bacteria, chemicals and pollutants that non-distilled water might contain. It also has the property of being able chelate out inorganic minerals out of the body.

Because there are no minerals in distilled water, take a multi-mineral supplement before you sleep. If the water you drink is not distilled, then make sure that you drink water purified with a reverse osmosis system. Reverse osmosis systems remove chlorine, bacteria and toxins. Because they also remove minerals, you must supplement your diet with multi-minerals, especially magnesium.

Important note: Avoid drinking water from plastic bottles. Research shows that water stored in plastic containers can be contaminated from a chemical that is harmful, especially when left in the heat.[29]

THE POWER OF JUICING

As we have discussed, vegetables and fruits are very alkalinizing, having an anti-inflammatory effect on the body. They also contain an abundance of enzymes and a variety of nutrients. When fruits or vegetables are juiced and consumed immediately, the nutrients and enzymes are quickly assimilated into the bloodstream. Juicing is a powerful way to cleanse your system, reduce inflammation and increase vitality levels. In addition, health-conscious people have used juicing to aid in healing chronic and serious diseases.

Drinking your own homemade vegetable juice is a more effective way to consume fresh enzymes and nutrients than ingesting them in pill form. When juiced, the nutrients are released and are assimilated faster and more thoroughly throughout your system than if you ate the vegetables.

Vegetable contains less sugar and is the better choice than fruit juice. However, do not drink too much vegetable juice as it might cause you to detoxify your system too quickly, leaving you feeling nauseous. I recommend drinking a maximum of one eight-ounce glass per day of freshly juiced vegetables. If you are on a detoxification program, you may have two juices per day.

Making your own juices does require a home juicing machine. There are many excellent juicers on the market. The differences lie in their price, function and in the ease cleaning after juicing. There are also "juice bars" in many cities now where you can order a fresh squeezed juice.

OPTIMUM TIMES TO JUICE

There is nothing better than starting your day with a fresh juice. You can feel the effects instantly. If you want a real vitality boost, substitute a fresh juice for your morning coffee. The juice will feed and nourish your system in a way that coffee cannot. If you must have something hot, substitute your morning coffee with hot water and freshly squeezed lemon.

It is best to consume fresh vegetable juice apart from meals. If you must eat them close to a meal, drink them first and wait 15 minutes before eating.

Mid-morning is a great time to have a vegetable juice of choice. Vegetable juices tend to build vitality and restore energy. Listed below are the various vegetables that can be juiced and their benefits. While you can juice any vegetable, I have listed the most common ones.

POWER VEGETABLES FOR JUICING

Carrot: Known for their high content of beta carotene, carrots contain various alkalinizing vitamins and minerals; must be used in moderation by those with blood sugar issues due to notable levels of natural sugars.

Beet: A helpful cleanser for the liver and gall bladder; contains many vitamins and minerals and a high level of iron, making it a blood strengthener; increases stamina; beet greens are rich in

Vitamin A and B-6, iron and calcium; very strong taste makes it best used in combination with other vegetables.

Cabbage: Is claimed to help heal ulcers, constipation and skin conditions; full of vitamins and minerals; in large quantities can cause bloating and gas—eight ounces or less should be sufficient.

Celery: Is high in sodium and minerals that are very relaxing to the system; reduces inflammation, lowers blood pressure, assists with insomnia, constipation, fluid retention; reportedly fights gout.

Cucumber: A natural diuretic, this juice has a very soothing effect and delicate taste. The peel is high in Vitamin A and should be included with juicing. It is a good source of Vitamin A, manganese and chlorophyll.

Ginger: A natural digestive aid, a small amount of this added to your juice gives it a tasty "kick". Ginger is a powerful anti-inflammatory. Avoid a week before surgery.

Garlic: Packing a powerful punch, small amounts of garlic, such as two cloves, acts as an antibiotic, bolsters the immune system, lowers blood pressure and has a cleansing effect. Do not use garlic within one week before surgery.

Spinach, Kale, Parsley and Dark Leafy Greens: These vegetables contain highly concentrated sources of minerals such as magnesium, iron, calcium and potassium as well as Vitamins K, C, B and E.

Apple: One of the only fruits you can add into a vegetable blend, apple is high in pectin. It sweetens the juice and contains Vitamin A, C, B-1, B-2, B-6 and various minerals. Use the peel if it is not waxed.

PREPARATION

I feel that it is always best to use organic fruits and vegetables, especially if you are drinking juice from root vegetables such as carrots and beets. Root vegetables absorb and filter their uptake of water through the roots; thus, if the soil is contaminated with pesticides, carrots, beets or turnip roots tend to absorb all the pesticides in a concentrated manner.

Always wash all vegetables and fruits with water whether or not they are organic. You can also use a brush along with a mild produce soap solution. If organic vegetables are not available to you, there are a number of bottled solutions meant to remove pesticide residues and bacteria. These are available in most health food stores. Alternatively, you can make your own with equal parts of white vinegar and water and soaking the produce for five to 10 minutes. You may scrub hard-skinned veggies with a brush and the solution.

THE RECOVER QUICKLY DETOXIFYING JUICE BLEND

3 to 5 carrots

½ small beet

3 large stalks celery

1 apple

A handful of spinach

1 tbsp. ginger

3 tbsp. parsley

1 peeled lemon

This blend is delicious as well as cleansing to your system.

THE MASTER CLEANSER

Those who are able to fast may try a gentle cleansing of the body using the Master Cleanser. It's best sipped throughout the day.

FAST FOR A DAY ON THE MASTER CLEANSER

If your surgeon approves, this fantastic cleanser is delicious and easy to make. It allows you to fast the day before your surgery (which you may need to do in many surgeries). It provides energy and has a mild cleansing effect on the body. Some people enjoy fasting on this cleanser for three to four days at a time.

Sip on the Master Cleanser throughout the day:

1 gallon of purified water	Mix together
The juice of 1 to 3 organic lemons	Drink the whole gallon in one day
4 tablespoons of real maple syrup	

This will assist you in the "cleaning-out process" as well as hydrate your body. It is very pleasant-tasting and usually provides enough energy to help you through your day. This can be a good substitute for caffeine drinks, sodas, salty consommé and sugary drinks. Shake before using.

Do not fast without physician approval.

❗ TAKE ACTION

Hydrate with 2 quarts of pure water daily.

Alkalize your system with organic, fresh vegetable juice.

Use Master Cleanser for a day or two prior to your surgery.

CHAPTER 6

NUTRITIONAL SUPPLEMENTS TO EXPEDITE YOUR RECOVERY

Always remember that the future comes one day at a time.

—Dean Acheson

Many types of surgeries deplete your body of specific vitamins and minerals. It is important to supplement those missing nutrients to support your recovery process.

The supplements listed below have been found to be the most effective for preparing for and recovering quickly from surgery. Everyone's surgery, health condition and circumstance is unique. Some of these supplements may or may not be appropriate for you so you must review this chapter with your surgeon and seek physician approval before taking them.

THE OPTIMUM SUPPLEMENT PROTOCOL FOR YOUR RAPID RECOVERY

1. **Proteolytic Enzymes** – Proteolytic enzymes may be the most single important supplement you can take before surgery. They are so important that many plastic surgeons routinely

recommend their patients use them before surgery. However, there are some physicians who are not informed about their ability to produce rapid healing in the body.

What Are Enzymes?

Enzymes may be the most important component of physiological life. Made from amino acids, an enzyme is an efficient catalyst for a specific chemical reaction and speeds that reaction up tremendously. There are more than 10,000 enzymes produced in the human body.

Proteolytic enzymes function to break down protein molecules in the body. Bromelain, papain, trypsin, chymotrypsin and pancreatin are some of these proteolytic enzymes that are naturally produced in small quantities in the pancreas and small intestine. As we age, the body's production of these essential enzymes slows, causing a need for supplementation. These same enzymes are found in plant sources such as papaya and pineapple. They can also be derived from animal and laboratory sources.

Supplemental proteolytic enzymes serve two different functions. The first is to aid in the further digestion of proteins, which begins in the stomach.

If proteolytic enzymes are taken apart from food, they pass directly into the bloodstream. Here they facilitate the removal of the metabolic waste products that occur in surgery and injuries. They serve to increase blood flow throughout the injured site, thus facilitating the flow of nutrients required for rapid healing. Proteolytic enzymes reduce inflammation by breaking down accumulated swelling, which, in turn, reduces pain at the site of the incision. The healing process of the incision is also accelerated, as is the overall healing time.

How They Affect Recovery

Proteolytic enzymes have been shown to reduce joint and muscle pain, improve circulation, improve the outcome of shingles and lower cholesterol levels. In addition, proteolytic enzymes appear to augment immune function as well as elimination. This assists in warding off infection at the site of a procedure.

Several studies show that proteolytic enzymes aid in recovery from surgery; the results showed reduced pain, inflammation, and swelling. A double-blind, placebo-controlled trial of 80 people undergoing knee surgery found that treatment with mixed proteolytic enzymes after surgery significantly improved rate of recovery, as measured by mobility and swelling.[30]

Dosage

Depending on your specific condition, dosages may vary. For many who are having surgery that is not complicated or risky, proteolytic enzymes are best taken in small doses three to four times per day. With physician approval, you might be able to take them for 10 to 14 days before surgery, ending three to five days before the procedure, unless your surgeon directs otherwise. They should be taken in-between meals or they will be utilized for digestion. The idea is to load them into the bloodstream in preparation for the surgical procedure.

As with every supplement, please check with your surgeon for approval before taking these supplements.

With a track record of more than 30 years, there are two prime enzyme formulations used worldwide by athletes and health care practitioners to accelerate recovery.

Wobenzyme N is one of the best known formulations. It is often available at local health food stores or may be purchased at our online store at www.recoverquicklyfromsurgery.com

Protease works in a broader range of pH and contains a blend of effective protein hydrolyzing enzymes. These must be

RECOVER QUICKLY FROM SURGERY

POSSIBLE SIDE EFFECTS OF PROTEOLYTIC ENZYME USE

If you are having a transplant surgery, you may want to limit their use to pre-surgery, as proteolytic enzymes enhance the immune system. This could *possibly* cause transplant rejection.

They *may* act as blood thinners. Most patients tolerate their use well up to the date of surgery.

If you are taking sedative drugs, consult your physician about taking bromelain.

In most cases, proteolytic enzymes may be used effectively right up to three days before surgery. Make sure you review the proposed use of these enzymes with your physician and/or healthcare provider to determine the dose appropriate for you.

purchased through a licensed health care practitioner or at our online store at www.recoverquicklyfromsurgery.com

2. Traumeel – This is the second most important supplement you will want to take before your surgery. It contains more than a dozen homeopathic remedies, making it the best complementary formulation for recovering quickly from surgery. It aids in tissue healing by reducing swelling and inflammation, while acting as an analgesic. While it most effective in acute injuries, it can be taken pre-surgically to aid in rapid healing. The best dose is one tablet taken five to 10 times a day without food.

3. Bioflavonoids – Bioflavonoids, derived from citrus fruit, have been documented to contain anti-inflammatory properties and may help reduce post-surgical swelling. A derivative from a naturally occurring bioflavonoid called rutin, when taken in pill form known as oxerutins, shows some evidence of reducing the swelling occurring after an operation. In one double-blind trial, researchers gave oxerutins for five days to 40 people recovering from minor surgery or other minor injuries, and found oxerutins significantly helpful in reducing swelling and discomfort.[31] Some supplements contain bioflavonoids, such as Vitamin C with bioflavonoids.

4. Key Vitamins for Healing – Surgery usually involves the use of anesthesia and other medications. These substances readily deplete the vitamins, minerals and specific antioxidants in the body, causing post-surgery fatigue and malaise. These vitamins are essential for the everyday functions of the human body, notably the immune system.

Sadly, many of the fruits and vegetables consumed today are lacking in proper amount of vitamins needed for optimum recovery. Therefore, it is essential that you supplement your body with a sufficient amount of these nutrients before your surgery. These may be taken individually or in a multivitamin available in both pill and liquid form. A reputable supplement company will guarantee the amounts shown on the label. You will want to consult your health care practitioner for a recommendation for a formula or purchase one from our online store.

Vitamins are best taken before noon with food.

Vitamin A. Known as an antioxidant as well as an immune booster, this vitamin is also helpful for healing skin wounds. It promotes collagen synthesis, which is needed for connective tissue repair.

Vitamin B. Vitamin B is an essential vitamin necessary for nerve function, metabolism, healthy skin and muscle tone, as well as preventing several forms of anemia. You may want take one additional Vitamin B-complex 100 with your multi-vitamin.

They are better taken with food.

Although B-vitamins help to relieve stress, they tend to be energizing. To avoid insomnia, take before noon.

Vitamin C. Also known as a powerful antioxidant, Vitamin C is essential for wound healing as well as enhancing the immune system. You may wish to take additional Vitamin C with your multi-formula. If you take too much Vitamin C, you may experience a loosening of the bowels. If you are taking blood thinners, ask your physician about Vitamin C.

Vitamin D. Called the sunshine vitamin, Vitamin D is noted for its power to maintain strong bones, muscles and nerves and for boosting the immune system.

Vitamin E. A superior antioxidant, this vitamin is an immune-enhancer with powerful anti-inflammatory properties. It assists with bruising and may also be placed around the edge of wounds after surgery to prevent scarring and the formation of keloids. Be sure to use d-alpha tocopherol or mixed tocopherols— the natural form of Vitamin E that is more potent. Because it acts as a blood thinner, discontinue all but small amounts for 10 days before your surgery.

You may also wish to take additional Vitamin B and C to manage any stress leading up to the surgery, as well as to enhance wound healing.

Consult your surgeon about taking supplements prior to surgery. While most are extremely safe, your doctor may recommend that you abstain from certain supplements.

5. **Essential Minerals for Healing** – Minerals can be taken in a

multi-formula, either in pill or liquid form. They may be included in your multivitamin formula in small amounts. Because surgery often involves skin, bone, muscles and joint healing, you may also want to take additional amounts of certain minerals that aid in healing. They are best taken before bedtime, as they are relaxing to the system.

Calcium. This important mineral is not only a bone builder, but is essential for proper nerve and muscle function and essential to the healing of muscle and bone. Protein interferes with the uptake of calcium into the bone, so it is best taken apart from meals or right before bed. There are several forms of calcium on the market, the best being calcium citrate/malate and calcium orotate, as they may have the greatest bioavailability.

Magnesium. Magnesium is important for the production of protein, the function of certain enzymes and energy production. It can help reduce pain by relaxing muscles post-surgery, as well as help you sleep more deeply. Useful for pre-surgery jitters, this excellent muscle relaxant also helps with post-surgical constipation.

Selenium. An essential trace mineral, selenium supports the immune system and helps prevent infection. (Selenium deficiency has been detected in post-surgical gastrointestinal patients.)

Zinc. Acting as an immune booster and an aid to wound healing, zinc is a powerful addition to pre- and post-surgical supplementation. It is essential for rapid wound healing. Check with your physician about using zinc while taking any antibiotics, amiloride, penicillamine, tetracycline, Warfarin or fluoroquinolone antibiotics.

Best Bet: Use a high quality multivitamin formula that encompasses many of these vitamins. Some vitamins or minerals, such as Vitamin C or zinc, may be taken apart in higher doses.

---

6. **Antioxidant Formula** – For any patient undergoing a prolonged surgery, I recommend that they take vitamins, minerals and supplements in the form of an antioxidant formula for one month before surgery, ending about ten days before their procedure. The formula should contain moderate amounts of Vitamin A, C, D and E, in addition to L-Glutathione, zinc, co-enzyme Q10 and selenium. Doing so can insure increased energy and well-being during the post-surgical recovery period.

7. **Probiotics** – Probiotics such as Lactobacillus Acidophilus and Bifidus are live microorganisms thought to be beneficial to the host organism. Because drugs administered during surgery may offset the balance of intestinal flora, taking a high quality probiotic before and after surgery is very helpful in maintaining the proper balance of intestinal flora, assisting in bowel function. The formula should contain 15 billion live organisms. The most effective ones are refrigerated.

   Be sure to take a probiotic after surgery if you receive antibiotics or steroids. This will help prevent a yeast overgrowth syndrome in the gut.

8. **Immune-Boosting Formula** – An immune-boosting formula is geared to assist you in fighting post-surgical infection if your system has been weakened by alcohol, drugs, cigarettes, anesthesia, stress, poor diet, previous bacterial infections or other illnesses. There are many products available that blend the ideal amounts of vitamins, minerals and probiotics to enhance your immune system.

Best Bet: Ideally the immune formula would contain small amounts of zinc, vitamins A, C, D3 and E, goldenseal, echinacea, bioflavonoids, probiotics and proteolytic enzymes. Stop taking any supplements with amounts of Vitamin E over 30 IU at least 10 days before your surgery.

9. **Key Amino Acids** – Clinical studies have shown that adding amino acids to one's diet may improve the healing process after surgery.[32] If you are depleted before going into surgery, you may want to take a formula with a variety of amino acids, or take them individually for specific results. For convenience, you can purchase a blend of amino acids. Below lists the types of amino acids that are helpful.

L-Arginine. This amino acid has been clinically reported to aid wound healing because, as a growth hormone releaser, it triggers the body to make protein. ***Note:*** *If you have a heart condition, seek the advice of your physician before taking.*

L-Cysteine. This sulfur-containing amino acid is an excellent adjunct to healing both internally and externally. It is necessary for collagen production, which makes it a powerful supplement for recovery from both burns and surgery. It works best taken with Vitamin E and selenium.

L-Glutamine. Surgery can be very taxing on your stores of L-Glutamine, an essential protein needed in the repair of muscle tissue thereby causing muscle deterioration. It is also very helpful for "leaky gut syndrome" and the autoimmune diseases that may arise from a poorly functioning intestine tract. Note: avoid taking if you have kidney or liver problems.

Best Bet: Try a high quality amino acid formula that contains the amino acids listed above.

10. Homeopathy to Augment Your Healing Process – According to the Society of Homeopaths, homeopathy is "a system of medicine which involves treating the individual with highly diluted substances, given mainly in tablet form, with the aim of triggering the body's natural system of healing."[33]

The following remedies are often used to treat pain and swelling in many parts of Europe and South America, as they have no known side effects.

Arnica 30c. Many complementary medicine practitioners suggest using arnica for the pain from swelling, lacerations, bruising and general trauma to an area. It is the main ingredient in Traumeel, which is more effective over a range of needs.

Hypericum 30c. Use Hypericum for nerve pain from either traumatized or inflamed nerves. Begin with Hypericum 30c then progress to Hypericum 200x if nerve pain persists.

Phosphorus 30c. Reduces the negative side effects of anesthesia and inhibits excessive bleeding. Take one tablet, four times per day for the week after surgery.

Carbo Veg 30c. A "must have" for all laparoscopic surgeries where surgeons inflate the abdomen with CO_2 gas. Use this remedy to reduce the side effect of the CO_2 gas which often refers pain into the right shoulder after laparoscopic surgeries. Take one tablet every 15 minutes until pain subsides or take one every few hours after surgery to prevent the pain from developing.

Staphysagria 200c. This remedy may be useful if there is mild post-operative internal bleeding, as in abdominal surgery. Place one tablet in a water bottle, sip throughout day. Take four to six doses until bleeding subsides. If bleeding persists, consult with your doctor.

Rescue Remedy. This specially prepared homeopathic tincture is formulated to treat shock and trauma incurred from accidents, injuries or emotional traumas. It may also be taken prior to surgery, as it will not interfere with any medications. This remedy is also is very helpful immediately after a surgical procedure to ease any persisting feeling of trauma.

Hepeel. This remedy is a formula that relieves nausea and abdominal discomfort as well as the referred shoulder pain from CO_2 gases used in laparoscopic surgery.

If unexpected ongoing pain persists beyond a reasonable time after your surgery, consult with your surgeon and/or complementary health care practitioners.

PROTOCOLS FOR JOINT SURGERIES

If you are an athlete having a sports-related joint surgery and you wish to optimize and accelerate your recovery, you may wish to use the following additional nutritional products.

1. **MSM (Methylsulfonylmethane)** – This compound is an excellent anti-inflammatory compound for joints, especially knees, hips and shoulders. Clinical trials involving osteoarthritis of the knee show that use of MSM significantly reduces pain and makes it easier to perform normal activities of daily life.[34]

   MSM is a naturally occurring nutrient found in small amounts in foods. It vitally supports the health of joints, skin, hair and cartilage. It promotes the growth of hair and nails and can be soothing to irritated skin. It can be taken by itself or in combination with other joint supplements such as chondroitin and glucosamine sulfate.

2. **Glucosamine and Chondroitin Sulfate** – These two sulfur-containing compounds are usually found together in supplement form. They are excellent anti-inflammatory agents and clinically have been found to reduce pain and help rebuild cartilage in joints. In surgeries involving the joints of extremities, it would be useful to take these in combination before and after surgery. I have found that a daily, consistent use of glucosamine produces positive results in accelerating healing and reducing joint pain.

Best Bet: I prefer and use Cosamin DS by Nutramax, as one of the highest quality formulas glucosamine sulfate.

Note: You may realize better results by taking these two supplements apart from meals. If you are diabetic, use under physician's care. Both may act as mild blood thinners as they reduce inflammation. Consult your surgeon before taking.

THE EIGHTY-NINE YEAR OLD GOLFER

An 89 year-old patient loved golf and played all his life. His game was impaired by hip and knee degeneration and accompanying pain. He began to take MSM and Cosamin DS. When he finally had a hip replacement, his recovery was extremely rapid for his age. He attributed his speedy recovery to taking MSM and Cosamin DS before the surgery.

QUICK GUIDE FOR NUTRITIONAL SUPPLEMENTATION

Below are general recommendations for adult dosages. *Because everyone's health issues, weight and age differ, always consult with your surgeon before taking these, especially if you have an illness such as cancer, kidney, heart or liver issues or if your surgery could be life threatening.* If your surgeon is not familiar with these supplements, I encourage you to utilize the guidance of a respected natural health care practitioner that understands the power of nutritional support before and after surgery. This individual could be another physician, chiropractor, a nutritionist, osteopath, acupuncturist or naturopath who is experienced in assisting patients with protocols for preparing for surgery with their surgeons. Together with your surgeon, your healthcare team can determine whether there are any health concerns or contraindications with taking the supplements and or dosages listed below. These dosages may be decreased or increased according to your primary health care professional's recommendations. I have found these to be an effective dosage for the average healthy individual with uncomplicated health issues.

Visit our online store at www.recoverquicklyfromsurgery.com for discounted pre- and post-surgical supplements that may accelerate your recovery.

Cosmetic Surgery

Wobenzyme N	3 tab/3x/day, Day 14 to Day 5 before surgery
Traumeel	5-10 tablets daily until day of surgery
Antioxidant Formula	Days 30 to 7 before surgery
Probiotic	3 doses 14 days before and then after surgery
Multi-Vitamin	1 dose AM
Multi-Mineral	1 dose PM
Rescue Remedy	1 to 10 doses, before and after surgery
Zinc	Take as directed. Be careful not to take too much as it can interfere with the absorption of other minerals.
Vitamin C	2000 mg a day
Bromelain	After at least seven days from surgery or as

physician recommends, take two times a day on an empty stomach. Do not take longer than 10 days consecutively.

Elective Joint Surgery

Wobenzyme N	3 tab/3x/day, Day 14 to Day 5 before surgery
Traumeel	5-10 tablets daily until day of surgery
Cosamin DS	3 capsules/day
Antioxidant Formula	Days 30 to 7 before surgery
Probiotic	3 doses 14 days before/after surgery
Multi-Vitamin	1 dose AM
Multi-Mineral	1 dose PM
Rescue Remedy	1-10 doses, before and after surgery

Back Surgery

Wobenzyme N	3 tab/3x/day, days 14-5 before surgery
Traumeel	5-10 tablets daily until day of surgery
Vitamin C	2000mg/day
Hypericum	1 tab 4-5x's/day for nerve pain and distress
Antioxidant Formula	Days 30 to 7 before surgery (if long surgery)
Probiotic	3 doses 14 days post surgery for antibiotic use

Laparoscopic Abdominal Surgery

Wobenzyme N	3 tab/3xs/day, Days 14 to 5 before surgery
Traumeel	5-10 tablets daily until day of surgery

Antioxidant Formula	Days 30 to 7 before surgery
Probiotic	3 doses 14 days before/after surgery
Multi-Vitamin	1 dose AM
Multi-Mineral	1 dose PM
Rescue Remedy	1 to 10 doses, before and after surgery
Phosphorus 30X	1 tablet, 4x's/day for anesthesia side-effects
Hepeel	1 tablet 4x's/day for shoulder pain from gas
Carbo Veg 30C	1 tablet post surgery, 4-5 x's/day

Pain Management

Rescue Remedy	4 doses /day or as needed
Traumeel Tablets	1/ hour, before and after surgery
Hepeel	1/hour, for post laparoscopic shoulder pain
Proteolytic Enzymes	2 tablets, 4 doses/day to reduce pain and swelling

WHERE TO GET THE RECOMMENDED SUPPLEMENTS AND FORMULAS:

Buy them at your health food store, from your health care practitioner or online at **www.recoverquicklyfromsurgery.com** .

FOODS AND SUPPLEMENTS TO AVOID BEFORE SURGERY

As mentioned, some foods and supplements have blood thinning effects, interact with medications or affect blood pressure. Some such as Valerian root may interact with anesthesia. Depending on the type of surgery and your health condition, these supplements should not be taken two weeks before surgery. A laparoscopic surgery, for example, may not be as invasive as other surgeries and may allow the use of these supplements closer to the time of your surgery.

Consult with your physician and health care provider about discontinuing the use of the foods and supplements listed below one to two weeks below surgery, especially if you are on blood thinners, as everyones' tolerances differ according to their medical condition.

NSAID's (Nonsteroidal anti inflammatory drugs)

Bromelain Discontinue use one week before surgery or earlier if your physician suggests.

Vitamin E

Chamomile

Devil's Claw

Ginkgo Biloba

Ginseng

Feverfew

Kava Kava

Licorice

St. John's Wart

Valerian

EPA-DHA (fish oils)

Warfarin (ask your doctor)

The nightshade family: tomatoes, potatoes, peppers, eggplant. Use of these foods may alter the affect of anesthesia.

Heavy use of garlic or ginger as it acts as a blood thinner.

Citrus fruits and pineapples may interfere with the efficacy of penicillin.

Cigarettes and nicotine patches should be discontinued one month or more prior to surgery for optimum incision healing.

❗ TAKE ACTION

Consult a health care practitioner to determine a proper supplement regime.

Take an antioxidant formula for one month prior to surgery, completing it 7–10 days prior to ameliorate the effects of anesthesia.

Take proteolytic enzymes and Traumeel for two weeks prior to surgery.

CHAPTER 7

ACUPUNCTURE: ACCELERATE HEALING, DECREASE PAIN

The part can never be well unless the whole is well.

—Plato

Before my surgery, my acupuncturist advised me to receive a special treatment developed for those about to undergo surgery. I found that the initial treatment and a series of post-surgical treatments were calming and instrumental to my fast recovery.

Acupuncture is renowned throughout the world for pain intervention, health intervention and for increasing vitality. It is a powerful adjunct to recovering quickly. The 5,000-year-old Chinese technique of inserting fine needles under the skin at specific points in the body historically has produced a significant reduction in chronic pain and illness for its patients, as well as relief for acute conditions. The Chinese have performed surgeries without anesthesia, using needles for pain control.

According to acupuncturists, pain and disease derive from energy blocks along the specific energetic pathways just under the surface the body. Fine acupuncture needles, when strategically inserted along these invisible pathways, release energetic blocks and relieve pain and symptoms. Acupuncture can treat many of the underlying causes behind diseases by increasing blood flow and drainage to affected areas. Clinical studies have determined that acupuncture may reduce a variety of symptoms, including cancer pain, as well as quell nausea and boost immunity.[35]

Scientific researchers have determined that acupuncture releases natural pain-relieving opioids. These neurotransmitters deliver signals that calm the sympathetic nervous system and release neurochemicals and hormones. This in turn relieves pain and stimulates the body's ability to heal.

ACUPUNCTURE CAN REDUCE YOUR NEED FOR PAIN MEDICATION

Acupuncture treatments are clinically shown to reduce the need for opioids such as morphine, a class of powerful and addictive pain medications that can cause serious side effects. Recent clinical trials have shown that "using acupuncture before and during surgery significantly reduces the level of pain and the amount of potent painkillers needed by patients after the surgery is over", according to Duke University Medical Center anesthesiologists who combined data from 15 small, randomized acupuncture clinical trials".[36]

More importantly, however, the study goes on to note, "While the amount of opioids needed for patients who received acupuncture was much lower than those who did not have acupuncture, the most important outcome for the patient is the reduction of the side effects associated with opioids". Tong Joo (T.J.) Gan, MD, a Duke anesthesiologist who presented the results of the analysis at the annual scientific conference of the American Society for Anesthesiology in San Francisco continues, "These side effects can negatively impact a patient's recovery from surgery and lengthen the time spent in the hospital."

Based on the results of this analysis, Gan recommends that

acupuncture should be considered a viable option for pain control in surgery patients. In addition, it has been shown to reduce risks of nausea, decrease itching and dizziness, as well as reduce cases of urinary retention.

You can ask friends for a referral to a seasoned acupuncturist in your locale. Since an acupuncture treatment can be extremely relaxing, patients often fall asleep on the table once the needles are placed. The needles rarely hurt upon insertion. Within minutes, its calming effect on the nervous system is experienced. Many patients feel renewed and restored, as if someone pushed a "reset button". Ask your acupuncturist if they know of pre-surgical protocols for either acupuncture or acupressure.

ACUPRESSURE

Acupressure is a non-invasive (no needles) alternative. In a study, UC Irvine anesthesiologists learned that acupressure treatments given to children undergoing anesthesia noticeably lowered their anxiety levels, making them and their families calmer.[37]

APPLYING ACUPRESSURE POINTS

There are several acu-points that are easy to locate to relieve physical pain as well as abdominal discomfort due to surgery. These are located on either the arm or leg and will be somewhat tender upon contact. You or your practitioner can apply gentle yet steady pressure for three to 10 minutes or until it the tenderness subsides.

Acu-point 1. Located on the inner wrist and aligned with the little finger, this point is helpful for anxiety, nervousness and fear.

Acu-point 2. Located one inch up and over from Acu-point 1 above, this point may relieve heart palpitations, anxiety and nausea.

Acu-point 3. Located in the middle of the crease of the inner elbow, this point may calm nerves and reduce anxiety.

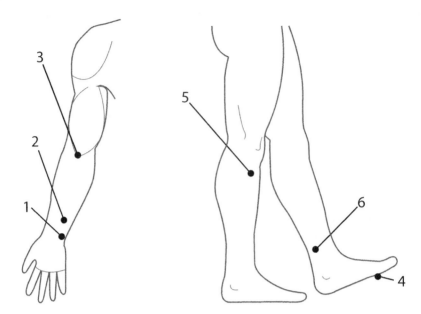

Acu-point 4. Located at the bottom of the ball of the foot, below the second and third toe, this point may relieve anxiety, diarrhea and insomnia.

Acu-point 5. Located in the fleshy part of the lateral shin muscle, one finger width lateral to the edge of the tibia and about a two-inch width down from bottom of knee cap. It is helpful in alleviating abdominal pain, distention, bloating and fatigue.

Acu-point 6. Located the width of four fingers above the tip of the inner ankle bone, this point can help to reduce insomnia, headaches, abdominal distention and pain. Do not use if pregnant.

❗ TAKE ACTION

Get an acupuncture treatment prior to surgery.

Practice using the acu-points prior to surgery.

CHAPTER 8
SLEEP TO RECOVER

Sleep is the best meditation.

—Dalai Lama

SLEEP: THE ULTIMATE RECOVERY TOOL

How many times have you woken up feeling better after a good night's sleep? Why is sleep such a critical component of any recovery process?

First and foremost, sleep removes us from the barrage of daily stimulus, giving the nervous system a chance to reboot. It also allows your body to "detoxify" ingested substances and pass them out of the body. Sleep allows your muscles and joints to mend and your cells to rejuvenate and rehydrate. Sleeping and dreaming also allows the psyche to process life stresses.

It is difficult to feel positive about anything if you are exhausted or tired. Fatigue can cast a cloud over your emotions. Getting enough sleep will assist you in boosting your physical stamina as well as managing day-to-day stress. Getting the right amount of sleep assists you in storing up the energy you will require to heal after your surgery.

15 SOURCES OF INSOMNIA

Stress is the most common cause of insomnia. It causes the release of cortisol, which signals your body to be awake and alert. Take time at the end of each day to decompress, especially by gentle exercise, swimming, yoga, a walk or deep breathing. Do your best to resolve your issues at the end of each day and affirm that the next day will bring a new perspective. You may want to draw a hot bath and drink an herbal sleep-inducing tea.

External Sources. Noisy neighbors, pets that need to be let out at night, late night phone calls and outdoor lighting are just some the external factors that can interfere with a full night's sleep. Make sure that you eliminate as many of these interruptions as possible.

Caffeine. Beware of drinking caffeinated drinks beyond the early afternoon as it can cause wakefulness into the night. Chocolate consumption can also cause insomnia.

Sugar. Consuming sugar can stimulate cortisol levels and cause wakefulness and insomnia. It is best avoided or consumed before 2 PM.

Alcohol. While it might initially induce sleepiness, it may cause an interruption in sleep, especially after midnight. If you must drink alcohol, consume plenty of water before bed to re-hydrate.

Late Night Eating. Eating late and going to bed on a full stomach can negatively impacting the quality of your sleep. Eating a heavy meal with glutens, such as wheat products, red meat, starches and sweets may also cause you to awaken with heartburn or an upset stomach. Instead of detoxifying, the body must work to digest food. If you go to bed by 10 PM, it is best to finish eating by 7 PM.

Low Blood Sugar. If you are hungry before bed or have low blood sugar issues, have a light snack such as ginger tea or a small piece of fruit or several almonds.

Hormones. As women age, declining levels of estrogen and progesterone may cause insomnia. If this is an issue, ask your gynecologist if a prescription for bio-identical hormones could help.

Exercise. Working out late in the evening may stimulate metabolism and cause wakefulness. For those who have insomnia issues, it is better to exercise in the morning or in the early evening.

Late Night TV or Computer Time. To insure a restful sleep, avoid being on the computer before bed, especially after 9 PM. Studies show that the computer screen emits low levels of radiation, that may disturb your nervous system. In addition, computer and TV screens emit a blue light, much like the daytime sky, which signals your pineal gland that it is time to be awake. Avoid watching television shows that are violent as this may cause an increase of adrenaline or cortisol, two hormones that inhibit sleep.

Bladder Issues. Drinking large amounts of fluids will cause you to awaken because of a full bladder, so it is best to limit fluid intake after 8 PM. Be sure to hydrate sufficiently during the day.

Hypoadrenia. The adrenal glands, located just above the kidneys, mediate stress in the body and are often overtaxed, causing restlessness and increased cortisol levels. Those who have adrenals that are depleted from poor eating habits and long-term stress may experience difficulty falling or staying asleep. Adrenal supplement are available and should be procured from your healthcare provider. Other glandular imbalances, such as hyperthyroidism, can cause sleeplessness as well, so be sure to consult with your health care provider if insomnia is an ongoing issue.

Late Night Bedtime Hour. Most people need between seven and 10 hours of sleep per night, with eight hours being the average. Some choose to stay up and then sleep in late. The hours you sleep before midnight offer the most potential for rejuvenation. According to Ayurvedic medicine, there is a natural sleep cycle from 10 PM to 6 PM, meaning a healthy hormonal system is wired to sleep well during these hours. If you stay up past 11 PM, there is a chance that you will override this cycle and find it difficult to go to sleep.

Irregular Bedtime Hours. It is also important to establish a regular bedtime. It is ideal to get eight hours of sleep if possible. Avoid taking naps, unless you have no trouble falling and staying asleep.

Medication-Induced Insomnia. If you are suffering from insomnia, ask your physician if any of your prescribed medications could be causing sleep disruption. Some over-the-counter medications contain caffeine. B vitamins are known to be stimulating, and herbs such as ginseng and green tea extract may cause insomnia.

RELAX TO SLEEP

In addition to avoiding the above causes of insomnia, it is important to create a relaxed state in which to fall asleep. Meditation and affirmation CDs are soothing and oftentimes aid in sleeping. Playing the recorded sound of waves, a brook or other nature sound throughout the night may help the brain drop into a deep sleep. There are also special recordings that are useful in promoting sound sleep.

Deep breathing or a warm bath before bed may also help you sleep. For some, reading is a healthy promoter of sleep.

EFFECTIVE NATURAL SLEEP SUPPLEMENTS

Below is a list of herbs, vitamins and minerals that can aid in sleep problems. These natural sleep aids should not interfere with surgery but you may review them with your doctor. You may find some or all of these combined in various formulas.

Natural Relaxants

Calcium	Vitamin B12
Trace Minerals	Lavender
Magnesium	Melatonin
Tryptophan	Kava
Passionflower	Valerian
Hops	Adrenal Calm
Chamomile	

If you have a chronic insomnia, talk to your physician or health care specialist about taking medication. There are some over-the-counter medications such as Unisom that may assist you in falling asleep if natural remedies are not effective. Ask your doctor if these are safe for you to take. Beware of certain prescription sleep medications as they may have serious side effects in some people.

If you are going to take an over-the-counter sleep medication, I recommend taking a small dose first and placing it under your tongue to let it dissolve and be absorbed directly into the bloodstream. This will allow you to take less medication to sleep. The less sleep medication you take the better, as there can be side effects such as dry skin, dehydration, drowsiness and itchy skin.

If you suffer from insomnia, do not rely on a medication to put you to sleep. It is important to attend to the other components necessary for deep, profound sleep to ensure a healthy and speedy recovery.

! TAKE ACTION

Commit to getting ample sleep.

Review the suggestions for good sleep and make one or more changes.

Preparing Emotionally for Surgery

And the day came when the risk to remain tight in a bud was more painful than the risk it took to blossom.

—Anaïs Nin

Facing surgery almost always involves encountering some level of stress, nervousness, fear or other uncomfortable emotion. Your surgery may invoke some intense feelings such as anger, frustration, sadness, fear, guilt or shame. Rather than ignore "uncomfortable" emotions, it is important to acknowledge your feelings to yourself and perhaps to someone who is close to you. Repressing these feelings can cause an underlying element of additional stress.

If there was ever a time to allow yourself to feel and express your feelings, it is at the time of your surgery. More than ever, you will need the support of friends and loved ones.

CAPITALIZE ON THE MIND-BODY CONNECTION

Ancient Chinese and Persian physicians understood that one's health can be negatively or positively affected by the deep connection between the mind and the body. They realized that a patient's mental outlook or beliefs have a profound effect on their physical body.

Clinical studies have proved that the mind-body connection is real and undisputed. One controlled, eight-week study monitored two groups. One meditated and the other did not. The ones who meditated briefly each day exhibited significant changes in their brain activity as measured by a EEG, or electroencephalogram. Their immune systems were shown to fight the flu vaccine with more force than the non-meditating group.[39] A series of other controlled studies indicated that meditation can enhance the immune system.[40] Additional research has concluded that negative emotions, such as stress and depression, can affect our physical health and lead to disease.[41]

Many years of clinical research demonstrates the interesting and definite connection between our mind and physical health. Studies indicate that patients given a placebo treatment, (a fake or dummy treatment often used for testing), will have a perceived or actual improvement in their medical conditions even though the placebo treatment should have no medical effect. For example, some patients in a controlled study might get the real treatment while other patients merely think they got the same treatment but actually did not. Researchers then compare the effects of the actual treatment with the fake or placebo treatment on the patients. This way, they can determine the effectiveness of the new drug and check for side effects.

STUDY: One study involving 180 individuals with arthritis needing knee surgery demonstrates this fact. Half of the patients received arthroscopic knee surgery and the other half received incisions, but only a fake knee surgery, as a placebo. The placebo surgery was just as successful as the real surgery.[42] The patients who did not actually have the full surgery believed they were actually having the surgery. The belief was enough to trigger brain responses that helped their knees to heal.

The emotional component may be the single most important factor in your recovery. Hundreds of clinical studies prove that the mind can direct the outcome of the body's healing process. Your emotional state can be the pivotal factor in the ease and speed of your recovery. It is not difficult to see this theory in action. Workaholics who maintain high levels of stress for prolonged periods of time are subject to heart attacks. Long periods of unexpressed fear or anxiety can suppress the immune system, causing infections or even cancer. Suppressed emotions can lead to high blood pressure, digestive complaints or inflammation in the body.

I encourage you to take an important step and connect with just what it is you are feeling about your surgery. Then employ one or more of the techniques listed below.

THE EFFECTS OF NEGATIVE EMOTIONS ON SURGERY

As noted, recent studies have shown that increased fear of outcome before a surgical procedure is associated with poorer outcomes, including longer hospital stays, more postoperative complications, and higher rates of readmission to a hospital. With this in mind, it becomes important to find outlets to express and release your emotions about your surgery.

ARE YOUR THOUGHTS HURTING YOU?

If you are wondering how you could determine if there are any emotional issues that may impede your accelerated recovery, here are some questions you may ask yourself:

Are you a person who tends to be fearful? Do you hold onto anger or resentment? Are you in a job or relationship that makes you unhappy or excessively stressed? Do you endlessly push yourself at work or in sports without taking care of your body? Do you feel disappointed in yourself that you have to have surgery?

If you answered, "yes" to any of these questions, you may be harboring stress or negative emotions that may inhibit your recovery. It can be difficult answering "yes" to any of these questions. However, gaining insight into these common life stressors may lead you to make changes that will accelerate your healing.

Interestingly, some hospitals are providing patients with brochures that suggest the importance of having a calm mind before surgery. With that in mind, utilize some of the suggested protocols in this chapter before your surgery to release the stress or negative feelings you may be facing. If it is difficult to do on your own, you may want to engage the help of a therapist, spiritual advisor or health professional.

RELEASING NEGATIVE EMOTIONS

If you are anxious and harboring negative emotions in your life or about your approaching surgery, it is important to find a way to "upgrade" your emotions to maintain a more positive state of mind. Here are some simple suggestions.

- Write your feelings in a journal. Be specific and honest—it is a safe place to "let it all out."

- Ask a trusted friend to be an "active listener". Their role is to listen to you without talking, interrupting or giving advice. Ask them for a succinct amount of time, usually 15 to 30 minutes, while you express your emotions directly with statements such as, "I am feeling scared", "I am really sad and worried." The goal is to allow yourself to express your feelings without having to explain them. Talking through these feelings, is a form of releasing them. This simple technique is powerful and often brings a sense of peace.

- Breathe deeply in and out. Imagine inhaling each breath with a sense of peace and thoughts of your surgery successfully completed, no pain and a 100 percent easy recovery. As you exhale, breathe out any fear or negative feelings. Actors, athletes and anyone who is under the stress of performing use this technique to augment their composure and inner peace.

- Find a counselor, therapist, clergyperson or spiritual advisor who will expertly assist you in talking through your feelings. I suggest a brief phone interview over the phone to determine if they are match for you.

AN EMOTIONAL CLEARING TECHNIQUE

In my clinic, I use this highly effective technique to assist my patients in releasing their emotions: by holding specific acupuncture points on the head while accessing the emotion, the conscious brain is able to process and release the emotion in a matter of minutes.

- Identify any negative emotions you are feeling.

- Place the index and middle fingers of each hand on both the left and right emotional points located on the forehead as illustrated.

- While holding these points, tune into your emotional issue or feelings by thinking about any negative feelings, (such as fear, dread, sadness, anger or anxiety), about your life or upcoming surgery.

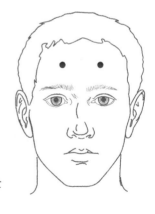

- Breathe deeply and stay connected to those feelings. There will be a moment you will spontaneously take in a deep breath and the feelings will release.

It is a simple, yet powerful and fast way to release layers of unwanted emotions.

AVOID NEGATIVE PEOPLE

It is important to surround yourself with those who are positive, supportive and reassuring. Refrain from giving details of your health to anyone who is a constant worrier or complainer. They will reflect their worry back to you and create more stress. Do not allow others' negativity affect your emotional state.

TAKE TIME TO PREPARE EMOTIONALLY

Often the need for surgery comes at inopportune times, creating a feeling of being stressed and overwhelmed. Even with elective surgeries, many patients will attempt to carry on with their day-to-day activities right up to the day of their surgery.

Are you always busy tending to your responsibilities? Are you feeling overburdened by constant caretaking of others? Do you neglect taking time to eat properly, sleep enough and have emotional downtime? Have you let yourself get run-down?

In the time leading up to your surgery, it is important to eliminate unnecessary distractions and obligations to take care of yourself in all ways. This will allow you to prepare yourself not only physically but emotionally. Recognizing the emotional and mental elements of surgery is indeed an important step in preparing to recover quickly.

IMPROVE YOUR MOOD WITH MUSIC

Music is used in film, public places, athletic events and even in the operating room to create a specific mood or feeling. Soothing or up-beat music can shift and uplift our negative feelings towards more positive feelings. If you find that you are stressed, distracted or fearful around the time of your surgery, dig into your music collection for songs that will bring you to a more positive frame of mind.

Find songs with a positive message that will filter into your subconscious mind. Sometimes, songs with no words, such as classical or ambient music, can uplift the emotions. Perhaps there are songs from your past that will always bring up a happy memory or create a positive feeling as you listen.

If you have an iPod or CD player, create a collection of songs that makes you feel good. Play it when you are in your car, exercising or having quiet time. If you have chosen ambient music, play it while you engage in creative visualization about the success of your surgery. This will allow your visualization to sink more deeply into the subconscious.

Many hospitals will allow you to listen to music before and during the surgery. It is best to ask the surgeon ahead of time about bringing your iPod and earphones into the surgical room.

EXPECT OPTIMUM RESULTS

To achieve optimum results using mind-body techniques, it is important to create an expectation for a speedy and complete recovery. If you talk to your surgeon about your expectations for the outcome of the surgery, he or she will then be able to clear up any misconceptions or fears that you may be harboring. This will also inspire trust in the upcoming procedure, and thereby enhance your expectations for a positive outcome. An optimistic attitude can do wonders for patients' recovery.

STUDY: Researchers reviewed 16 studies spanning 30 years, analyzing patients' attitudes after surgery. The review appears in the August issue of *Canadian Medical Association Journal*. "In each case the better a patient's expectations about how they would do after surgery or some health procedure, the better they did," said author Donald Cole, of the Institute for Work and Health in Toronto. Patients who were scared or pessimistic about their recovery did not recover as quickly as the optimists, or as well. Those with more positive expectation had less pain.[44]

BECOMING AWARE OF THOUGHTS AND REDIRECTING THEM

Most people have thousands of thoughts each day. Most of them are unconscious, negative, fear-based or project into the future or the past. In most cases, thoughts emerge from our subconscious response to the stresses of life. It takes focus and energy to remember to engage in uplifting thoughts during of your waking hours.

Why bother watching and changing your thoughts? Thoughts create feelings. Engage in angry or sad thoughts and watch your mood change. The same is true for positive thoughts. Positive thoughts not only make you feel better, they replace the unconscious negative thoughts and feelings you may be generating about your condition. Fearful thoughts cannot coexist with happier, more positive ones.

Many of us do not realize that we can *choose* our thoughts. You do not have to be a prisoner to negative thoughts or allow them to affect your emotions. Your beliefs are simply a thought you hold to be true. The more you practice redirecting your thoughts to more positive, empowering ones, the sooner your negative thinking patterns and fear will systematically dissipate.

With this in mind, it is critical for those seeking optimum results to actively choose positive thoughts in preparation for their healing process. While it is important to acknowledge the stress and emotions in our lives for the purpose of releasing them, it is equally, if not more important, to focus on positive or uplifting thoughts and feelings.

Monitor your thoughts and redirect negative ones. Empowering thoughts and feelings will not only help you accelerate your healing, they are an important part of maintaining physical and emotional health *after* surgery.

One of my patients, who had cancer, utilized positive affirmations daily in order to release her pervasive pain and fear. She always reached for more positive thoughts rather than engage with the fear of succumbing to her cancer.

You can focus your thoughts towards health with these suggestions:

- Stay present to what you are experiencing and breathe – you may find relief and increased clarity.

- Find something to be grateful for every day, even if you are suffering and in pain.

- Choose one empowering thought and repeat it constantly out loud or to yourself daily.

- Despite the severity of your health issue, try to determine the silver lining in your health issue and approaching surgery.

THE PACT

One of my students sent me a patient who had read about my work and desired a session. When I first saw her in the waiting room, I was taken aback by how emaciated her body was. This patient explained to me that she wanted some emotional and energetic healing for the cancer that she had been battling for over seven years.

In our process together, we discovered that she had unconsciously made an agreement to have cancer when she was only 19. A beloved uncle was dying of cancer and she stated, with all her heart, that she wished she could have cancer instead of him. He died shortly thereafter and she forgot about her comment, which when she had uttered with commitment, created a kind of psychic "contract".

Years later, we discovered this "pact" she had made and knew that it was time to undo her wish for cancer and the related, subconscious negative thoughts she had carried for years. After 15 minutes of work, she released this pact. We both experienced a shift in energy. She thanked me and said that she would like to see me again. I intuitively knew that I would not see her again and hoped that it would not be because the cancer had taken her.

Six weeks later, she emailed me a joyous letter that her cancer was in remission and she was out of pain. She shared that was moving across the country to be reunited with her family. She noted that she was feeling wonderful and thanked me for her healing. Her release of the subconscious negative thoughts around the pact had freed her.

FIND THE LESSON

Each test or challenge in your life offers you an opportunity to grow. You must discern the nature of the lesson being presented by your current physical condition, and then do your best to resolve your issues. Often this recognition will prevent a need for future medical intervention. Find the lesson if you can. It will liberate you in a new way.

Perhaps there is no lesson to be learned and your condition is due to an accident, a genetic or environmental factor. In three decades of practice, however, I have found that there is usually some underlying emotion or life pattern linked with many of my patient's conditions. With some reflection and insight, many patients realize what the correlating stressors to their condition are.

THE MIRACLE OF LAUGHTER

Norman Cousins, a former editor of *The Saturday Review*, revitalized a popular belief in the power of laughter and humor in his book *Anatomy Of An Illness* (Norton, 1979). Cousins recounted his own self-healing experienced in 1964.

Since then others have utilized laughter and humor to ameliorate pain and emotional suffering. Watching comedies and uplifting movies while recovering may be the simplest and best way to apply this modality of emotional healing.

THE ART OF RECEIVING

So often, we attempt to accomplish the difficult tasks in our life alone. We do not want to burden others or appear vulnerable or incompetent. Some people are so used to giving to others that they forget how to receive; they do not know how to ask for help. Others will routinely deny the help offered by others out of habit or conditioning.

If ever there was a time to allow others to help you, it is now. It is human nature to want to help others. Many of your friends will be eager to assist you in some way during your surgery, especially if you will be bedridden for any length of time.

Reach out to those friends and loved ones who you know will want to help you. If you are not used to allowing others to help you with emotional support, this will be an important opportunity to leave your comfort zone. Let loved ones and friends bring you cheer, humor and companionship.

Your surgery will have an effect on those close to you. Understand that the process of your surgery is part of their journey too. Convert your experience from "my surgery" to "our experience in this together". It will shift the immediate feelings of vulnerability and isolation to the positive feelings of support and love throughout your surgical experience.

THE POWER OF PRAYER

Do not discount the power of prayer, whether you are praying for yourself or if others are praying for you. Ask your loved ones and your community to pray for a successful, easy surgery. At the very minimum, it is comforting to know that your loved ones are holding you in their thoughts.

Studies show that the power of prayer or positive support is definitive:

- Elderly individuals who rarely went to church had a higher stroke rate than those that went regularly.

- Heart patients that did not participate in a religion had a much higher chance of death after surgery.

- Hospitalized patients who never attended church stayed in the hospital three times as long.[45]

❗ TAKE ACTION

Check in daily about your feelings surrounding the surgery.

Listen to uplifting music and breathe deeply.

Ask for support from a close friend.

Watch a comedy and laugh out loud.

Choose a positive thought about your surgery, and then repeat often.

Ask your friends or church group to keep you in their prayers.

CHAPTER 10

THE BODY-MIND CONNECTION AND SURGERY

You need to learn how to select your thoughts just the same way you select your clothes every day. This is a power you can cultivate. If you want to control things in your life so bad, work on the mind. That's the only thing you should be trying to control.

——Elizabeth Gilbert, *Eat, Pray, Love*

Once we recognize our negative thoughts and the disempowering emotions they create, we can change our emotional state by choosing to think positive, affirming thoughts. Many of the great entrepreneurs and athletes of our time used positive thinking and creative visualization to manifest their empires and to excel at new levels. You can use the same techniques to accelerate your recovery process.

EMPOWER YOUR HEALING PROCESS WITH AFFIRMATIONS

An *affirmation* is a proclamation spoken out loud or silently that presents a positive outcome. The use of positive affirmations has proven to be extremely effective for many purposes including reducing pain and shifting negative emotions, as well as improving general health and state of mind.

Stating an affirmation repeatedly and with conviction trains the subconscious mind to register it as truth. You literally program your subconscious mind to believe that your upcoming surgical experience has already happened and was safe, easy and painless, with a positive outcome. You do this by stating that your positive outcome has *already occurred*. If done correctly, the subconscious mind does not know the difference between the stated *now* and the *imminent future*.

This does more than allay fear. Scientific studies show that outcomes greatly improve with positive beliefs and expectations. Increasingly, research is showing that the mind has the power to influence the outcome of medical procedures through intention, visualization and focus.[46]

MAXIMIZING THE POWER OF AFFIRMATIONS

1. Affirmations can affirm that you are ready to heal on all levels.

   "I am open to healing on all levels".

2. Affirmations can help attract the things into your life that you need to heal.

   " I am attracting the perfect surgeon and the resources necessary to completely heal easily and quickly".

3. Affirmations may also be spoken by friends and loved ones on your behalf. This is operates like prayer, and is very powerful when two or more speak it as a truth.

   "We know that Mary heals completely and painlessly each day."

4. Affirmations can be repeated while walking or exercising. If you align your affirmations with the rhythm of your exercise workout, they will settle more deeply into your subconscious.

   "My body is getting stronger and healthier every day".

5. Joyfully affirm your gratitude for the expected optimum results, as if it has already occurred.

"I give thanks for the great success of my surgery!"

HOW TO CREATE EFFECTIVE AFFIRMATIONS

According to Steven Covey, a world-renowned writer and speaker in the personal development field, affirmations are most effective if you:

- make them about you;

- state them in the positive;

- state your outcome in the present moment, as if it has already manifested;

- create a clear picture to accompany them; this augments your subconscious mind's belief that your affirmation is truth;

- energize your affirmation with positive feelings, even if you have to muster them up.

Emotions drive the affirmation into the subconscious mind to create a new belief. Try to affirm with joy and conviction. If you are in pain, ill or very frightened, try to remember the most significant past memories when you felt elated and happy about something. Bring those thoughts to mind and overlap those thoughts with your affirmations until they blend and merge.

Repeat your affirmation until you feel a shift in energy or attitude. You might notice the shift in a few minutes or it might take a few days. Change the words of the affirmations to suit your situation. You may experience an initial feeling of resistance or find them unbelievable. This initial resistance is normal. Over time, you will integrate them into your subconscious mind. The more you practice any suitable affirmation, the sooner you will experience a positive outcome.

EMPOWERING AFFIRMATIONS

I am completely healthy and happy with my new, improved physical condition.

My body is relaxed and ready to heal quickly.

My body is stronger and healthier each day.

I am enjoying my rapid healing process.

I am loved by my friends and family. Their love and good wishes cause instant and fast healing.

I let go of all the things that I cannot control.

I am surrounded by love. I am completely safe.

My hospital stay is filled with loving energy from the prayers of my family and friends.

The Divine lovingly guides my doctors during my operation.

My surgeon is caring, competent and is helping to restore my body to perfect health.

I release the past and know that all is well now.

My surgery is an incredible success. My body and mind are renewed.

My body easily and readily releases all forms of disease, swelling and toxins.

My medication helps me heal.

PRACTICING AFFIRMATIONS

Do what premier athletes all over the world do to accelerate their healing process. Use the power of the mind to accelerate your healing with the following suggestions.

- Place your written affirmations where you will remember to say them.

- Write your affirmations in a journal, 30 times for 30 days.

- Record them on your phone or on a CD, and/or play them as you go to sleep.

- Say them out loud whenever you have a moment, especially if you are having negative thoughts about yourself or your upcoming surgery.

- Speak your affirmations with enthusiasm and gusto, as if you are already observing the positive results.

- To deeply embed an affirmation into your subconscious, repeat it while your relax, with eyes closed, 30 to 100 times.

- As you use affirmations, you may need to change them to reflect your evolving goals. You might feel bolder in your declaration as you gain confidence in your ability to influence the outcome of your surgery and recovery process.

MEDITATION TO ACCELERATE THE HEALING PROCESS

There is a vast body of clinical research concluding that meditation can positively prepare you for surgery and reduce pain thereafter. Meditation has been scientifically proven to alter and improve your physiology, immune system and mental acuity.[47]

In several controlled studies, meditation and guided imagery were shown to lower cortisol levels and thus control pain, as well as reduce bleeding during surgery.[48] According to Ohio State University Medical Center's Dr. Hari Sharma, "Meditation has been shown in one study to produce significant increases in left-sided anterior brain activity, which is associated with positive emotional states. Moreover, in this same study, meditation was associated with increases in antibody titers to influenza vaccine, suggesting potential linkages among meditation, positive emotional states, localized brain responses and improved immune function."[49]

Numerous studies further indicate that meditation can significantly reduce pain, stress and anxiety before and after surgical and medical procedures.[50]

SELF-GENERATED MEDITATION PRACTICES

There are many ways to meditate. Many meditators generate their own meditation or "practice". Others listen to pre-recorded guided meditations. Here are common ones practiced all over the world.

Technique #1. With eyes closed, inhale slowly and evenly. Pause at the top of the breath. Notice your thoughts. Release the breath evenly as you release your thoughts. Repeat this process continuously for 10 minutes. Even if your mind wanders, bring it back to observing the breath. Release thoughts as you notice them. Increase your meditation time as you are able.

Technique #2. Choose one word as a mantra. Words such as love or peace are powerful mantras. Some meditators use universal sounds such as OM or HUM. Replace your thoughts with this word, repeated over and over, thereby disrupting the flow of unconscious thoughts or negative self-talk. With practice, your mind will shut off and you will enter into a state of awareness that is conducive to healing. This state of "no-mind" is extremely beneficial to the nervous system, as well as instrumental in relieving stress.

Technique #3. While walking in nature, follow the breath, noticing the colors and sounds of your environment. Keep focused on the breath, and notice the natural elements around you.

GUIDED MEDITATION

Overall, a practice of guided meditation before, during and after your operation has been proven to:

- lessen pain levels
- reduce recovery time (thus shortening your hospital stay)
- strengthen your immune system
- allow you to sleep more deeply
- reduce the use (and thereby the cost) of pain medication.[51]

CREATIVE VISUALIZATION

While meditation on its own is a powerful tool in calming and stilling the mind to enhance healing, creative visualization utilizes the power of the mind to see, feel, sense and experience an outcome before it happens. There are many recent studies proving that performing creative visualization (sometimes referred to as "guided imagery") before and after surgery can reduce pain and speed up recovery time. Studies show that patients who completed a guided imagery program had a shorter average length of stay in the hospital, as well as lowered pain medication costs.[52]

Neuroscience and sports psychology theorists maintain that by visualizing an outcome repeatedly, the mind can prepare the body more favorably to consciously desired outcomes.[53] After listening to the guided visualizations in the weeks preceding your surgery, your subconscious mind will begin to create positive pathways or associations with them. You may then want to play these in an iPod or similar device during your surgery to enhance the outcome.

Many professional athletes employ creative visualization before their games. They visualize their moves and shots being successful, energized and precise. They feel each success in their body, relishing the exaltation of winning. They mentally rehearse the critical moments of victory, prepared for the endurance required not only of their body but also their mind.

A powerful way to direct your thoughts is to visualize your surgery going smoothly and painlessly with a full recovery. Put on some soothing music and visualize your surgeon effortlessly performing the surgery. Remember, those well educated about their surgery tend to enjoy better outcomes, so have your doctor educate you about the details of your surgery. Use that knowledge to imagine in detail what will happen, adding in thoughts such as "there is barely any bleeding and no pain," and "my body is already beginning to heal as the surgeon works."

As with performing affirmations, the most important aspect of creative visualization is to actively use all of the senses to anticipate desired outcomes. If you are well educated about your surgery, you can practice anticipating the positive outcome of the surgery in a hopeful or excited state. See the actual surgery happening step-by-step, with a painless recovery period and the desired outcome nothing short of miraculous.

TIPS FOR EFFECTIVE CREATIVE VISUALIZATION

Visualize a positive outcome as if it is happening now. Studies show that your subconscious may not know the difference between the imagined surgery and an actual surgery. If you can see and feel that the surgery has been a complete success, your body's physiology will respond accordingly, accelerating the healing process. In addition, if your subconscious already registers that the surgery was a success, you will see a reduction in pre-surgery fear and anxiety. This alone will improve post-surgical outcomes.

Use positive emotions to empower your creative visualizations. Generate excitement when you visualize your recovery process and your brain will reward you by creating the necessary chemicals for the desired results. Imagine being ecstatic at the lack of post-surgical pain. Visualize an optimum timeline for healing and imagine feeling amazed at how quickly you recover. See and feel yourself surpassing your expectations of health and well-being, and you will make your surgery one of the more positive experiences of your life.

Ask your surgeon to explain your upcoming procedure in as much detail as you can handle. After educating yourself about the details of your surgery, use this information to visualize your surgeon performing the procedure with expertise and confidence. Imagine hearing the surgeon comment how well the operation is going. Imagine feeling an upbeat tone in the operating room. See the surgeons, anesthesiologists and nurses happy and working together as a team. You may also visualize a divine source guiding the surgeon's hands during the surgery.

Visualize often. Visualize positive outcomes several times a day. It is similar to working and developing a muscle—the more you exercise it, the more it develops. Include visualizing minimal bleeding, with little discomfort or pain. The more you visualize an easy, painless surgical outcome,

> I once fell off a horse onto my lower back. This injury prevented me from being able to do my normal running workout for weeks and weeks. How did I heal the injury? One day I saw someone running in my neighborhood. I felt how much I wanted to run again, so I went home, closed my eyes and vividly visualized myself running with no pain. Two days later, the injury mysteriously healed and I went back to my workout the next day.

the more you will increase your chances of sending conscious and subconscious messages to your brain to manifest this outcome.

Imagine your future. Imagine yourself pain-free, fully recovered and very happy– as if it is happening in the present moment. Imagine a feeling of freedom and a new lease on life. Imagine yourself relaxed and energized. Get excited about things you will do *after* your recovery and visualize them as happening now. See yourself doing them with your loved ones.

Visualize out loud. Describe the desired healing process out loud to yourself or another person as if it is happening in the present moment. Include key points about the surgeon's precision, imagining diminished post-surgical pain and a rapid recovery period. Include any positive feelings you can muster, such as hope, excitement, peace or joy.

Friends and family can also visualize for you. Ask your friends and family to visualize a positive outcome with an easy, painless recovery. Give them specifics to visualize, such as time of surgery and desired timeline of recovery. Discourage worrying; encourage them to think happy thoughts for you. Emphasize that you are having surgery to make your life better.

Create the perfect visualization recording. Many phones now have recording devices on them. Make your own custom guided visualization recording of your voice describing all procedures of the surgery going perfectly, and state your positive affirmations. Play the recording in the car, before going to sleep, when doing mundane chores (mowing the lawn, laundry, etc) to implant it in your subconscious mind.

Use recorded guided imagery during surgery. If you are not able to create one of your own, guided imagery visualizations may be found on CDs, podcasts or on other electronic download formats. (You may go to www.recoverquicklyfromsurgery.com to download guided visualizations.) Many hospitals recognize the power of guided imagery and allow their patients to wear headphones in the operating room during their procedure. It will relax you and assist your subconscious mind in preparing for the most positive outcome after surgery. Clinical research proves that there is some evidence of patients' awareness during surgery, even under anesthesia. Ask your surgeon if you can bring in a portable CD or MP3 player such as an iPod with headphones, and play the recorded meditation during your procedure. Begin listening to a guided imagery audio before your surgery and ensure that it is long enough to run throughout. If it is a long procedure, you will want to put it on continuous play.

Ask the staff ahead of time to allow the recording to continue while you are in the recovery room. Some family members may opt to listen to your guided meditation as well, to relieve their anxiety relating to your surgery.

RECOVER QUICKLY THROUGH HYPNOSIS

Sometimes it is more effective to allow a professional to input helpful suggestions into the subconscious through the practice of hypnosis. Using a series of visualizations and suggestions, the hypnotherapist induces a state of high suggestibility. In this relaxed state, hypnotic suggestions penetrate deeply into the mind without distraction, allowing the mind to focus more deeply on the process of healing quickly and painlessly. The hypnotherapist uses safe and specific techniques to bring the subject into a deep state that allows enhanced receptivity to positive suggestions regarding their healing.

Many clinical studies show that hypnosis has been highly effective in reducing pain. In one recent study, women who underwent brief hypnosis immediately before their breast lumpectomies or biopsies required one third less sedative medication during their procedure. Patients reported that their post-procedure experiences were also significantly improved when they used hypnosis. They reported a decrease in intensity of pain, nausea, fatigue, discomfort and emotional upset as well as perception of pain compared to the non-hypnosis group undergoing similar procedures.[54]

Research shows a varied use of hypnosis in the medical field. It can be used to reduce recovery time, pain and anxiety. One study showed that patients who received hypnosis healed faster (about two months ahead of the non-hypnosis group).[55] Hypnosis has been used in some cases when anesthesia was not tolerated. It has also been used to reduce the perception of pain in cancer patients, breast surgery, child labor and other surgeries. Another study of chronically ill patients found a 113 percent increase in pain tolerance among highly hypnotizable subjects versus those who were not hypnotized.[56]

Hypnosis is effective in a way similar to creative visualization. At the very least, if you are nervous or dreading surgery, one or two sessions of hypnosis may be very beneficial.

! TAKE ACTION

Write down several positive affirmations and place them on your mirror. Repeat several times a day out loud.

Listen to soothing music and visualize your surgery going perfectly.

Meditate daily.

Quiet the mind and end with a positive thought.

Make your own recording of affirmation on your phone- listen to it daily.

Seek the help of a hypnotherapist to create a CD with positive imagery.

CHAPTER 11

PAIN: WHAT TO EXPECT

Life shrinks or expands in proportion to one's courage.

—Anaïs Nin

Patients often undertake surgery with the hope and expectation to be pain free after their surgery. Yet most surgeries involve post-surgical pain, which is often the most challenging aspect of the surgical procedure.

Being educated about post-surgical pain will prevent you from being discouraged about the results. By learning what levels of pain to expect, you can prepare emotionally and mentally. This will allow you to be more positive during your healing process, thus accelerating the healing time.

It is important that the surgeon manage your expectations. Be sure to ask your surgeon what type of pain most patients experience for your specific surgery. Many of my patients were very disappointed with their surgeries because they did not expect to have the high levels of post-procedure pain. It is important to be informed about the quantity and quality of post-surgical pain to expect–and how long you will have to endure it.

Studies show that patients who better educate themselves about their surgery in advance experience less pain and heal faster.[57] If you mentally prepare yourself for pain and discomfort you will fare better in enduring it.

ASK YOUR SURGEON IN ADVANCE

Have your surgeon create a pain management plan with you in advance, reviewing all of your options. It is necessary to accurately follow your surgeon's advice, especially if you are having a major procedure. You do not want your pain level to exceed a moderate threshold, as it will inhibit the healing process.

To aid in this process, you should inquire about the details of your proposed prescriptions with the following questions.

- How long should you expect to experience pain from your procedure?

- What kind of pain is typical for this kind of surgery on a scale from one to 10?

- How many medications will be required?

- Will you need an anti-coagulant (blood thinner)?

- Will new medications conflict with current required medications?

- What is the timetable for their use ?

- Can you drive while taking these medications?

- Are any of the medications opioids?

- Are any of the medications addictive?

- What are their side effects, if any?

Some pain medications innately have effects similar to opium and can be addictive. Some of these are hydrocodone (Vicodin), Meperidine (includes brand name Demerol), morphine (includes MS Contin), Oxycodone (includes brand name of Oxycontin), codeine and Ambien. Ambien is designed to help you sleep but it has been misused and is highly addictive. Pain medications may block natural processes in the body that reduce inflammation. Because inflammation can create pain, it is beneficial to quit taking these medications as soon as possible.[58]

ADDICTION

If you have or have had an addiction to drugs or alcohol, you might want to discuss this with your surgeon, especially if that addiction relates to proposed pain medications. Former addiction to drugs may make you less responsive to pain medication and require more to get the same effect. You may also want a management plan to wean off the prescribed medication.

If you feel that you are becoming addicted to any pain medication, contact your physician immediately. An addiction can occur without a patient realizing it, so do not be ashamed if you feel this is happening. It may be too difficult and sometimes dangerous to wean off a medication by yourself. Thus, do not delay in getting assistance from your physician as soon as you become aware of an addiction problem.

INFORM YOUR DOCTOR

You know your body's needs and proclivities the best. Disclose to your physician or surgeon all of your current prescription drugs, over-the-counter medicine, whether you are taking insulin and all nutritional supplements to make sure they will not interfere with your pain medication or anesthesia.

Tell your surgeon about any reactions to medication you have experienced in the past. If you have had procedures before, inform your physician which pain medications worked best. Let your doctor know if someone in your family has had a negative reaction to a drug being prescribed. These measures could prevent setbacks in your recovery.

You may wish to discuss your tolerance to pain with your doctor. Let them know in advance that you are willing to endure a mild to moderate amount of pain in order to ingest less medication. If you have a low pain tolerance or a high tolerance to medication, you may need extra medication.

If you are going to require a stay at the hospital, inform your doctor and hospital staff of any known food intolerances or allergies. While in the hospital, make sure you choose the healthiest food available on the menu and avoid inflammatory foods if possible.

Most importantly, informing your physician about any unique issues you have or have experienced in the past will only help them to select options for you that will be the safest and most effective. Don't be shy about asking about the magnitude of pain typical for your kind of surgery. Prepare yourself with this advance knowledge and then visualize your results surpassing your surgeon's expectations.

In addition, there may be side effects to medication, such as itchiness, nausea or constipation. If you experience these, inform your add doctor or nurse immediately, as there are ways to treat these temporary symptoms.

MANAGING YOUR PAIN

Pain medication is often a critical aspect of recovery. A body that is in pain is stressed and will recover more slowly. If you properly manage your pain, you will feel better, as well as be able to use other pain management techniques sooner, (such as deep breathing exercises). I do not discourage my patients from using prescription or over-the-counter medication as prescribed by their physician. Although some pain medications are highly addictive and toxic to your system, the appropriate medication is essential for mediating post-surgical pain and its stress on your body. However, the goal is then to get off the pain medication as soon as possible.

PRECAUTIONS WHEN USING PAIN MEDICATION

- Do not drink alcohol while taking pain medication.

- Take pain medication with food.

- Take only those medications prescribed by your physician.

- Tell your surgeon about other medications taken for health issues.

- Use fiber supplements and drink two to three quarts of water to offset constipation.

Fortunately, there are pain management protocols that can reduce the amount of medication needed as well as the amount of time it will be necessary. By implementing an anti-inflammatory diet, the recommended nutritional protocols described in this book – along with utilizing deep breathing and other pain mediating treatments such as laser treatments, acupuncture, acupressure, physical therapy, chiropractic and massage therapy – you may greatly reduce your need for pain medication.

In addition, you may reduce associated side effects and the length of time you require medication. Remember that meditation, deep breathing and hypnosis are known to reduce pain. Distractions such as watching TV, listening to favorite music or having visitors, may also lesson the perception of pain.

A PLAN FOR PAIN: NON-TRADITIONAL PAIN MANAGEMENT

According to a 2010 study in the *Journal of Patient Safety*, non-traditional therapies relieve pain among a wide range of hospitalized patients by as much as 50 percent.[59] The study shows that the implementation of inpatient integrative therapies, similar to those outlined in this book reduced self-reported pain by more than 50 percent, without placing patients at increased risk of adverse effects. "We struggle to provide effective pain control while trying to avoid the adverse effects of opioid medications, such as respiratory depression, nausea, constipation, dizziness and falls," says Gregory Plotnikoff, MD, one of the study's authors and hospital's medical directors. The treatments included non-pharmaceutical services: mind-body therapies to elicit the relaxation response, hypnosis, use of the TENS unit (Transcutaneous Electrical Nerve Stimulation), physical therapy, acupuncture, massage therapy, chiropractic, music therapy, biofeedback and more.

ESSENTIAL NATURAL PAIN RELIEF SUPPLEMENTS

Before your surgery, purchase these specific homeopathic remedies and bring to the hospital. Because they are homeopathic, there are no none side effects or contradictions to these remedies. Ask your nurse to give them to you after surgery:

Traumeel

Arnica

Hepeel

These natural pain relievers are known to be effective in reducing pain and the need for prolonged pain medication. (This information is more thoroughly covered in the preceding Chapter Six regarding nutritional supplements.)

Continued use of **proteolytic enzymes** can reduce post-surgical swelling and inflammation and thus relieve a source of pain. They should be taken on an empty stomach several times a day, with physician approval.

As soon as your doctor allows, begin taking the supplement protocols offered under Pain Management in Chapter Six. Implementing the recommended protocols before your surgery will decrease both the amount of pain medication needed as well as the length of time it will be required.

10 EFFECTIVE PAIN MANAGEMENT TREATMENTS

There is significant research showing that many natural methods alleviate pain while complementing the effectiveness of prescribed pain medication, thereby reducing the need for these drugs over time. Acquaint yourself with these methods before your surgery to facilitate your recovery and decrease pain levels as well as the need for prolonged medication.

1. Acupuncture. Perhaps one of the most powerful complementary pain management techniques available, acupuncture has been clinically proven to help in the recovery process and speed healing. Patients who received acupuncture as part of their pain management have showed significant drops in pain scores.

2. Physical Therapy. Most hospitals utilize physical therapy to assist patients in their healing process, reduce pain and mobilize joints that have undergone surgery. Some hospitals may offer extended rehab programs during a patient's hospital stay.

3. TENS. TENS is the acronym for Transcutaneous Electrical Nerve Stimulation. It is a small, portable, battery-operated device that sends mild electrical impulses to certain parts of the body to block pain signals from being transmitted to the brain. Use of the TENS may raise the level of natural painkillers called endorphins.

4. Cold Laser Treatment. The cold laser machine, a recent development in pain therapy, is being used for pain reduction, wound healing, bruising, swelling and immune function. Using either a diode ray or an LED emission, the laser penetrates the skin, increasing cell metabolism, detoxification and rejuvenation. It can also be used to minimize formation of external and internal scars. Sessions last three to 15 minutes and are administered by medical and chiropractic doctors.

5. Hydrotherapy and Ice Packs. Ice packs reduce inflammation and help mediate pain. Powered icing machines, such as *Cryo Cuff*, *Breg*, *Don-Joy* and *Game Ready*, provide continuous cold and compression to areas such as knees, shoulders and other extremities that have undergone a procedure, and may aid in reducing swelling, decreasing pain and accelerating recovery time.

6. Hypnosis. As mentioned earlier, hypnosis, which works with the subconscious mind, has been proven clinically to reduce pain. There are numerous ways to work with your subconscious mind in reducing pain, either by yourself or with a licensed hypnotherapist, as covered in the Mind-Body chapter.

7. Infratonic Machine. This technology has been used on patients to eliminate and reduce severe and chronic pain. The machine uses ultra low sound wave frequencies as an acoustical therapeutic massage device, deeply penetrating the injured area and relieving pain. Studies indicate that this instrument reduces swelling and pain in racehorses.

8. Continue the Recover Quickly Diet. This diet will minimize the amount of inflammation that occurs immediately after a surgery and assist you in your rapid and complete recovery. Less inflammation also means less pain, as the chemicals released in inflammatory states also register as pain factors. Avoid wheat, products, dairy, alcohol, caffeine and red meat. Eat primarily alkalinizing foods, with protein, as outlined in Chapter Four.

9. Acupressure. Acupressure uses pressure on specific acupuncture points to reduce pain. The points will be tender if they need treatment, and will decrease in tenderness with applied pressure for one minute up to seven minutes. Use the points outlined in the earlier chapter.

10.Biofeedback. Biofeedback uses monitoring devices to furnish information about autonomic body functions, such as heart rate or blood pressure, to the user, in an attempt to gain some voluntary control over that function. May be used for pain control.

MUSIC THERAPY

Music therapy is often used in hospitals to reduce pain, boost patients' moods, fight depression, reduce anxiety and fear, relax the nervous system, and facilitate deeper sleep. Clinical studies indicate that patients who listened to music as a means of post-operative pain management had a lower systolic blood pressure and heart rate, and required less oral pain medications.[60]

BREATH THERAPY

One of the oldest and most natural forms of pain control is engaging in deep breathing. Zen meditation practitioners and yogis alike have used breathing to control pain for centuries.

Do not underestimate the breath's ability to effectively manage pain. Consider the millions of mothers who use the Lamaze Method, the renowned pain technique involving slow, deep breathing to manage the pain of childbirth without medication.

Pain medication blocks the message of the pain in the brain; breathing through the pain releases it. Studies show that controlled breathing at a slower rate can significantly reduce feelings of pain, possibly by having a direct effect on the nervous system.[61]

If your health issue does not involve your chest or lungs, and you can breathe deeply without hurting the area of incision, you will find that deep breathing can greatly reduce pain, or at least help you cope with it. Breath work helps your body to relax and decreases anxiety.

There are several breathing techniques that will mediate pain. Practice any of the following techniques to breathe through pre-surgery jitters.

1. Yogic Breathing

Yogic breathing has been used for centuries to regulate blood pressure, increase oxygen in the lungs and reduce pain.

- Sit or recline in a comfortable position. Inhale slowing and deeply through your nose for a count of four. Pause and then exhale for six seconds very slowly, allowing the air to move across the back of your throat and through the nose, making a sound like "haaahhhhhhhh". Pause and repeat over several minutes.

2. Deep Breathing

This breath is very helpful for releasing pain and relaxing the body.

- Sit or recline in a comfortable position. Breathe in through your nose slowly, imaging that you are breathing into the pain, allowing the rib cage to expand to its full capacity.

- When you cannot inhale any more air, pause for one to five seconds, then release the breath through the nose, with control, over 10 seconds. Imagine you are releasing the pain as you exhale. Repeat for 10 to 15 minutes.

3. Stress Releasing Breath

This breath is very good for releasing stress, sadness or fear.

- Breathe in evenly through the nose. Pause.

- Exhale quickly through the mouth, sighing "Haaaaaahhhh" as you release the breath.

> If emotions should arise while you are performing any of the breathing techniques, breath into them and release them with the exhale. Allow yourself that opportunity to cry, laugh or yell…it is very therapeutic and often releases pain at the same time.

- Repeat, increasing the sigh in both length and sound until you feel a release of stress or a sense of peace.

TAKE IT EASY

To avoid a relapse in pain or a recovery setback, don't try to resume normal activities or jump back into doing chores too soon, even if you feel okay. Give yourself more time than you think you need.

! TAKE ACTION

Choose several alternate pain therapies to implement after surgery.

Plan to use Traumeel and other homeopathic remedies along with your pain medication.

Practice breathing techniques prior to surgery.

CHAPTER 12
DETOXIFYING FROM MEDICATION

Half the modern drugs could well be thrown out the window, except that the birds might eat them.

—Martin H. Fischer

Although necessary for surgery, anesthesia, pain medication, antibiotics, anti-nausea medication and opiates can tax the liver and congest the lymphatic system. This will adversely affect your healing and recovery time. Patients often experience malaise, headaches, fatigue, irritability and any variety of symptoms well after the surgery is over and they have completed taking their medication.

Recent studies have shown that patients who underwent surgery under anesthesia showed a suppression of immune function.[62] Because surgery takes a toll on the immune system, it will need support in eliminating the residue of anesthesia and all other medications. Anesthesia also depletes anti-oxidants therefore it is wise to take an antioxidant formula prior to surgery. In addition, the liver must process the anesthesia as well as other medications, so it too, needs support.

It is advised to allow prescribed medications to do their job, before you undertake your cleanse. It is best to detoxify gently and not while you are still taking strong pain medication. You may become ill, and experience flu-like symptoms, nausea and headaches if you detoxify too much or too soon. Generally, it is advised to wait at least two-three weeks after surgery or until you cease taking prescription pain or other medications.

With physician approval, and depending on the nature of your illness, injury and type of surgery, use any of the gentle cleanses offered below to eliminate the residue of anesthesia and pain medication. It is advisable to seek assistance of a natural health care provider who is experienced in assisting patients with detoxification if your surgeon or physician is not.

11 GENTLE CLEANSING OPTIONS

1. Water. Drink lots of purified water with or without the juice of organic lemons throughout the day. It is one of the best, most gentle forms of cleansing. Water should be consumed at room temperature and should not be tap water.

2. Vegetable Juicing. Drink one glass a day of freshly made juice made from fresh, raw, organic vegetables. A popular and effective blend of carrot, beet, celery, ginger, parsley and lemon is known to detoxify the liver, gall bladder and lymph. You will need a juicer or a Vitamix to prepare these juices.

If you are unfamiliar with the effects of juicing, begin with five ounces for a week or so, gradually increasing the amount to 16 ounces daily maximum. Drink your juice slowly, ideally first thing in the morning. You may then follow it up with

TIP! If you have a Vitamix or powerful blender, you may blend a drink of a half-cup of each of the following: apple juice, kale, cilantro, parsley, spinach and finely chopped celery. Add pure water, a peeled lemon and a small amount of ginger to aid in detoxification.

a detoxifying tea. Discontinue juicing if you feel nauseous or experience headaches. Be sure to drink plenty of pure water throughout the day. You may increase the amount of juice if you are experiencing positive effects.

3. Detoxifying Tea. You can purchase teas at your local health food store that include an array of herbs that gently detoxify your system and blood. Follow the instructions for the amount to use. One to two cups a day over a two-week period should assist in cleansing and restoring the healthy functioning of your organs and lymphatic system.

4. Diet. Following a healthy eating regime that emphasizes vegetables, low fat protein and healthy fat and carbohydrates will provide a suitable detoxification for most people. Consume small amounts of protein three to five times a day with cooked and raw vegetables. Add "good" carbohydrates in the form of whole grains and fruits, and small amounts of fats such as olive, coconut and canola oil. Continue to follow the Recover Quickly Diet for optimum results.

5. Antioxidant Formula. There are a number of high quality antioxidant formulas that effectively ameliorate the effects of anesthesia and prescription drugs. The formula should contain vitamins A, C, E, EFAs as well as selenium and zinc.

6. Herbal Tinctures. Silymarin, also known as milk thistle, has been used to protect and detoxify the liver. You may place the tincture directly under the tongue for maximum absorption or in a cup of cool or hot water. In most preparations it may be taken three times per day. Red clover is an effective blood purifier and may be used three times daily.

7. Bowel Cleanser. Once toxins leave the liver, they must be excreted through the bowel. You will want to use a good bowel cleanser that contains psyllium seeds, herbs and Vitamin C. Purchase a fiber-based product such as Perfect 7 or the Ultimate Cleanse, both which are gentle and contain fiber and herbal mixtures. Consult your health care professional for a recommendation for the proper product for you.

8. Sweating and Exercise. Sweating will quickly flush toxins from the lymphatic system. If you are unable to exercise, use a sauna or steam room for five to 10 minutes to promote lymphatic cleansing. To prevent dehydration, make sure you hydrate with purified water containing electrolytes. When you are able to continue exercising, wear heavier clothes to encourage sweating.

9. Lymphatic Massage. If your body is able to tolerate a massage without disturbing or hurting the injured area, it is one of the fastest ways to dislodge toxins in your body. Be sure to drink at least three glasses of water within three hours following your massage to flush out the dislodged toxins. You may also dry brush your skin and follow with a hot shower.

10. Epsom Salts Bath. Epsom salt is used to extract acidic wastes such as uric acid and other toxins out through the skin. If you are able to bathe, place one and a half cups of Epsom salts in a tub of comfortably hot water and soak for 15 to 20 minutes.

11. Homeopathic Detoxification Kits. Three homeopathic remedies, Nux Vomica, Berberis, and Lymphomyosot, taken together, offer a gentle detoxification process for lymph and bowel. Thirty drops of each are placed in a water bottle and sipped throughout the day.

Please visit our online store at www.recoverquicklyfromsurgery.

com if you are unable to find these and other recommended supplements in your local health food store.

! TAKE ACTION

Drink plenty of water, post surgery.

Take soothing Epsom salt baths.

Continue with antioxidant formulas if your procedure lasted more than one hour.

Choose a gentle detoxification program if you do not feel you are recovering quickly after several weeks post surgery.

CHAPTER 13

Preventing Scarring

*Scars show us where we have been, they
do not dictate where we are going.*

—David Rossi

With every operation, there is the potential for scarring. Your propensity to scar depends on the size and depth of your incision, your age, race, genetic tendency to scar and your health condition. Some surgical scarring can be very small and hardly noticeable, as in the case with small, slit incisions made arthroscopically. However, in other surgeries, incisions can be long and deep, with the potential to be disfiguring.

To minimize scarring, you must reduce inflammation, lower the risk of infection and protect the incision in its healing process. How well your scar mends may also be an indicator of how well you are healing internally. There are a half-dozen proven natural protocols that will inhibit scarring, though these therapies may not work for everyone.

If your incision is large and/or disfiguring, you may want to consult with a cosmetic surgeon. They are highly skilled in reducing scarring through their suturing techniques.

PREVENTING INFECTION TO THE WOUND

If your incision becomes infected, there is a greater chance of scarring. Observe your incision for the days following your surgery to check for any signs of infection such as redness, increased pain around the area of the incision or drainage of a cloudy or green fluid from the wound.

- Be sure to protect against infection by keeping the area clean and properly bandaged. Make sure you wash your hands before caring for the wound or changing the dressing.

- Be sure to change bandages as directed. You may need to prevent it from getting wet, so ask your doctor about optimum care for your incision. Keeping it dry and properly bandaged will help it heal quickly.

- Call your doctor immediately if you develop a temperature above 101 degrees or red streaking around the area.

- Smoking is known to cause of post-surgical infections, so it is important to quit before your surgery. Allergies, diabetes and obesity can also increase your risk of infections forming.

- Avoid shaving with a razor near the site of the surgery as razors can irritate your skin and make it more prone to infection. If the area needs to be shaved, special clippers will be used.

- Make sure that all healthcare providers who examine your incision wash their hands before touching you. Do not allow family and friends to touch the wound until it is completely healed. You may wish to ask them to wash their hands before they visit you, especially in the hospital.

Most surgical sites can be treated with either oral or topical antibiotics. Your doctor will determine if antibiotic treatment is necessary either pre-surgically or post-procedure.

COMMON TYPES OF SCARS

Typical Scars may heal with or without inflammation and swelling. There is usually a scab that forms and then, if left alone, falls off when the incision is completely healed. These scars are vulnerable to darkening if exposed to sunlight. It is important to apply an effective sunblock over your incision to prevent this darkening process.

Keloids are scars that are raised, thickened and often discolored. They form as the scar is healing and often continue growing. Some patients are prone to keloid formation due to genetics, race or body chemistry. In addition to diet and supplements, the use of laser and cosmetic surgery can reduce keloid formation.

Adhesions are fibrous threads or bands of tissues that form internally wherever there is trauma or injury to an area within the body, as in the case of surgery. Often, adhesions form between conjoining organs or internal structures. These adhesive fibers can thicken with age and pull on the connective and organ tissues, causing pain and disfigurement. Common places for adhesions are in the abdominal cavity, pelvis and heart. It is very easy for fibrous material to form between the colon or reproductive organs and the apron of tissue that connects to the colon.

If you are having a second surgery in the same site, your surgeon may encounter adhesions. Post-surgical infection or inflammation is often the cause of adhesions, and may make a surgery more difficult and more prone to complications. Most surgeons will do their best to clean up adhesions at the affected site. Because adhesions can be a source of pain well beyond the surgery, as well as causing future organ dysfunction, it is important to prevent adhesions when possible by reducing the possibility of infection or inflammation to the site.

PRE-SURGERY PROTOCOLS

If you are concerned about future scarring, it is wise to safeguard against infection and inflammation. Promoting a healthy immune system before your surgery can be facilitated with supplements and diet. Following the Recover Quickly Diet will bolster the immune system as well as discourage an inflammatory response. Taking the recommended supplements for wound healing before the surgery will have a marked effect on how fast and how well your scar heals. These include:

- **Vitamin A**- essential for proper wound healing;

- **Zinc** – essential for tissue repair via collagen production as well as wound healing;

- **Colostrum** – has a number of healing properties, one of which is wound healing;

- **Proteolytic Enzymes** –reduces swelling, thereby promoting wound healing;

- **Silica 30x** – homeopathic remedy that promotes wound healing;

- **MSM** – promotes healthy skin and wound healing.

HEAL YOUR INCISION, PREVENT SCARRING

- **Reduce Inflammation.** Swelling and inflammation may occur at the site of the incision. Use ice over affected area as directed by your physician.

- **Blood Flow.** After your incision has healed, if swelling remains you may alternate heat and ice at five-minute intervals.

- **Diet.** Continue following the Recover Quickly Diet.

- **Supplements.** Follow a nutritional protocol recommended in this section or by your healthcare practitioner. Utilize supplements such as zinc, Vitamin C and a scar cream if your physician approves.

- **Smoking.** Do not smoke before or after your surgery. Many plastic surgeons will not perform surgery on those who are smoking because of the deleterious effect it can have on healing the skin.

- **Alcohol.** Keep alcohol consumption to a minimum while you are in the healing process. Alcohol causes systemic inflammation.

- **Sunblock.** Keep your scar out of sunlight, as ultraviolet rays can darken scars. Use sunblock or clothing that is an effective sunblock when outdoors to avoid discoloration.

- **Topical Scar Creams.** Do not apply topical remedies until the incision has formed a solid scab. Then apply topical substances to the outside edges of the scab that interface with the undisturbed skin.

- **Protect the Incision.** Avoid putting too much stress on or stretching skin near the wound area. Once the wound starts to heal and all sutures are removed, you can massage the area gently around the wound to stimulate blood flow.

- **Silicone Sheets.** Some plastic surgeons recommend using silicone-based scar treatment sheets. These sheets help the scar to soften and fade over time.

EARLY CARE FOR INCISIONS

Immediately following surgery, it is important that you do not disrupt healing of an incision. First and foremost, you will want to protect it from infection by keeping it dry and covered. After four or five days it is often helpful to allow it some airflow so that the wound will scab. As soon as possible, or within two days, you may dab a small amount of aloe vera gel around the wounds. Aloe is very soothing and known to have beneficial effect on skin healing.

If the wound appears red, overly tender or "angry," or if there is pus forming internally or externally, you may first apply an over-the-counter topical antibiotic cream. If the area under the incision continues to swell, is hot or appears infected, consult your doctor.

If after one week the incision appears to be healing, begin dabbing Vitamin E on the outer edges of the scab. By waiting a week, you allow the skin to heal from inside out. If applied too early, the outer skin can heal over too quickly, not allowing the inner aspect of the wound to heal properly. Vitamin E use can be continued for eight to 10 weeks, depending on the severity of the scar.

EFFECTIVE SCAR-REDUCING THERAPIES

1. Cold Laser Treatments. Cold lasers can be extremely effective in promoting wound healing thereby reducing scarring. Most cold lasers penetrate up to five centimeters to provide a source of healing below the skin. You can do a Google search to see which chiropractors or other health practitioners in your area have a cold laser device. Consult with the practitioner in your area about your type of surgery and incision to see if cold laser therapy will reduce the effects of scarring after your surgery.

Treatment may require three to five applications a week for three minutes per treatment. Each cold laser therapy application offers immediate results by decreasing redness, swelling and bruising.

2. Topical Applications for Wound Healing

Vitamin E. Vitamin E can be used topically for softening the edges of a scab once a wound has started to heal. Although there are some studies refuting earlier claims about the effectiveness of Vitamin E, many find it to be soothing, as well as helpful in minimizing scarring.

Aloe Vera. This substance may be soothing to any redness around your incision. It also helps promote skin cell growth when used topically.

Manuka Honey. Biochemist Dr. Peter Molan of New Zealand has determined that Manuka honey from New Zealand heals wounds. This is attributed primarily to a natural non-peroxide antibacterial activity called UMF (Unique Manuka Factor). Proponents claim that using the honey topically and orally can accelerate wound healing.

Scar Gel. Scar creams and other silicone-based gels have been formulated to reduce scarring. The best scar creams are those that are gel or serum-based and use medical-grade silicone as their sole primary active ingredient. Visit www.recoverquicklyfromsurgery.com to purchase one.

Traumeel. Use this highly effective cream to reduce pain and redness around the incision area. It helps to reduce swelling and bruising.

3. Acupuncture. Acupuncture successfully can reduce scarring.

An acupuncturist can thread the scar with very thin, long acupuncture needles to restore the proper energy flow through the affected areas. Scars crossing meridians can have a detrimental effect on the body's energy system.

4. **Massage For Adhesions.** Scars are often located on top of areas of adhesions. Once a scar is completely healed, you may massage the area around it if you feel there might be adhesions forming. A knowledgeable healthcare practitioner such as a chiropractor, massage therapist or naturopath can perform a specific adhesion-clearing procedure. It may require several treatments.

THE PSYCHOLOGICAL EFFECT IN SCARRING

Understandably, large scars can have a psychological effect on the patient. If you have negative feelings about a scar, the trauma that caused it or anything related to the illness or injury that caused the need for surgery, then it might be beneficial to seek counseling regarding these issues.

! TAKE ACTION

If you tend to scar, procure anti-scarring cream.

Review all scar prevention procedures and choose appropriate treatments.

CHAPTER 14

SUMMARY:
KEY PREPARATIONS

Give me six hours to chop down a tree and I will
spend the first four sharpening the axe.

—Abraham Lincoln

It is ideal to prepare for your surgery for at least one month prior to your procedure. Hopefully, you have followed the suggestions about diet, exercise and lifestyle. You are now ready to implement supplement and as well as all other protocols outlined in the preceding chapters. There are four aspects in your preparations to recover quickly from your surgery.

Immunity. Your immune system will have an important part to play in your recovery by keeping you free from infection. It also assists in wound healing. It is ideal to promote a healthy immune system before surgery. If you develop a cold or the flu, you will not be able to undergo surgery.

Antioxidants. If you are undergoing a surgery that takes longer than one hour, your antioxidants are in danger of being depleted by the anesthesia. It is advisable to take an antioxidant formula, instead of taking many individual supplements.

Inflammation. Inflammation causes pain and swelling. Swelling by itself can also be a source of pain and discomfort. The

149

recommended anti-inflammatory supplements or remedies can be safely taken with pain medication and augment pain control. Several of these supplements may be taken before surgery to reduce post-surgical inflammation.

Recovery. Certain supplements and procedures will accelerate aspects of your recovery, resulting in less pain and need for medication.

ONE MONTH BEFORE SURGERY

- Improve fitness levels.

- Follow the Recover Quickly Diet.

- Get detailed information about your surgery.

- Often visualize your surgery going extremely well.

- Get as much sleep as possible; rest to store up reserves.

- Get your affairs in order.

Follow the RQFS supplement regime. Refer back to Chapter Six on supplements for specific recommendations, then obtain the advice of a healthcare practitioner for proper dosage of these supplements. You may also present the RQFS recommendations to your doctor for feedback. Use high quality supplements, preferably from a qualified practitioner or from the Recover Quickly Store at www.recoverquicklyfromsurgery.com.

Here is a list of the essential supplements that are clinically proven to enhance and accelerate your recovery from a surgical procedure.

- Antioxidant Formula
- Immune Boosting Formula
- Multivitamin with B-100 complex

- Multi-mineral
- Calcium/Magnesium Formula
- Time Release Vitamin C
- Essential Fatty Acids (Fish and Flax Seed Oil)

Your physician will usually inquire about medications and supplements you are taking. You will be asked to stop taking Vitamin E and EFAs 10–14 days before your surgery, as they are blood thinners. Be prepared to get a second opinion if your physician discourages you from taking any supplements more than two weeks ahead of your surgery.

Take vitamins early in the day with food. Take minerals later in the day with dinner or before bed. Essential Fatty Acids may be taken before bed.

TWO WEEKS BEFORE SURGERY

Follow the recommendations in Chapter Six for using the most effective supplements to accelerate your recovery. Take seven-14 days before your surgery, unless your surgeon recommends otherwise.

Proteolytic Enzyme Formulas such as:

- Transformation Enzyme Protease (containing bromelain, papain, trypsin, pancreatin, chymotrypsin.)

- Wobenzyme N.

    Dosage: Take five to 10 during the day, in-between meals or as directed by your doctor.

Consult with your physician about the use of enzymes, especially if you are undergoing chemotherapy or organ or tissue transplant. Enzymes also may decrease the effectiveness of anticoagulant medicines such as Warfarin or increase the absorption of tetracycline or amoxicillin.

151

Homeopathic Remedies

- Traumeel tablets or
- Arnica 30 X tablets
- Hepeel tablets if on several medications

Dosage: Take 1 tablet, six to eight times a day, separately from food, for two weeks prior to your procedure.

For the best results, create a calendar and note what to take each day. Take only if approved by your physician or alternative care doctor. *Consult with your natural health care specialist for proper dosage for your specific surgery.*

UTILIZING THE RECOVER QUICKLY DIET

Most physicians will not make any nutritional or dietary recommendations. You may wish to consult an alternative practitioner for specific information for your procedure and health status. Follow the Recover Quickly Diet for the weeks preceding your surgery.

After reviewing this diet with your health team and physician, per Chapter Four, you could:

- Eliminate or reduce red meat, alcohol, dairy, wheat, coffee, salt and sugar for two to four weeks. If you eliminate coffee, please take five days to wean yourself off it so that you do not develop a headache.

- Increase your consumption of alkalinizing foods, namely fruits and vegetables, up to 70 to 80 percent of your diet. Eat some vegetables raw, as they will have additional vitamins. Add protein to vegetable meals. Eat fruit by itself, in-between meals.

- Consume freshly made mixed vegetable juice to include carrot, beet, ginger and celery. You may also enjoy wheatgrass, kale, spinach, parsley and other greens. Enjoy with a squeeze of lemon. This will help you alkalinize and balance your system while gently detoxifying it. Do not drink too much raw juice per day. One glass a day should suffice.

- Strictly avoid salty, starchy, processed and fried foods. Avoid cured meats and salty cheeses.

- Avoid junk food such as candy, cakes, pies, chips, French fries, sugary drinks, sodas, ice cream, fast foods and foods with MSG, preservatives and pesticides.

- Increase your water consumption to two quarts per day, preferably in-between meals. Squeeze lemon in half of your water to alkalize your body. It provides a mild cleansing action.

REST AND SLEEP

Prepare for your surgery by getting ample rest and sleep in the weeks leading up to it. Don't leave preparations until the last moment. If you have time before your surgery, take some quiet time and visualize your procedure going exceedingly well, with optimum results.

THE DAY BEFORE YOUR SURGERY

A day or two before surgery your physician may order preliminary tests. Below is a list of suggestions that will better prepare your body for a faster surgical recovery.

- **Nourish yourself.** Drink freshly-pressed vegetable juice throughout the day.

- **Hydrate.** Drink two quarts of water throughout the day.

- **Traumeel, Rescue Remedy.** Take these and other recommended homeopathic remedies, as they will not interfere with your procedure.

- **Eat lightly.** Consume a clear soup with some protein and vegetables such as chicken soup with vegetables, and perhaps add some brown rice.

- **Foods to avoid:** Bullions, as most are high in sodium, which can cause inflammation. Sherbet, gelatin and some juices are high in sugar and corn syrup, which can cause inflammation. Coffee and tea are stimulants, which are best to avoid before surgery.

- **Fast from food.** Drink the Master Cleanser for energy if you need to fast for the whole day before. Consider drinking herbal teas, clear organic apple juice and clear organic chicken broth.

- **Fast from liquids.** You may need to stop consuming all liquids the night before, usually by midnight.

- **Cleanse the bowel.** With certain surgeries, your physician may also ask you to take a laxative, which will have specific instructions. The doctor will either give this to you, or give you a prescription so you can pick it up from your local pharmacy. Plan to spend four to five hours both taking it and being close to a bathroom.

- **Choose relaxing activities.** Email your friends with an update before the procedure and ask for their thoughts and prayers. Complete any tasks that may cause your stress and worry while you are recovering.

- **Sleep.** Plan to get at least eight hours the night before your surgery. Listen to relaxing music while you drift off to sleep. Affirm a positive experience awaits you.

While the actual surgery may not be in your control, your ability to prepare your body for optimum health beforehand will have a significant impact on your recovery time and pain levels.

WHAT TO PACK FOR THE HOSPITAL

Many surgeries are outpatient surgeries, meaning that patients will go home the same day as the surgery. If you will require a hospital stay of one night or longer, you will need to pack for the days you will be there. Here is an ideal list of what to pack:

toothbrush, toothpaste, brush, shampoo, deodorant
_____

pajamas, slippers and robe
_____

complete change of clothes
_____

slippers
_____

feminine products
_____

shaving materials
_____

day clothes
_____

reading glasses or, if applicable, contact lenses and cleaner
_____

medications and supplements for recovery as mentioned in this book
_____

healthy snacks
_____

music, iPod
_____

laptop
_____

books, magazines
_____

money
_____

cell phone and charger
_____

❗ TAKE ACTION

Download the appropriate questions to ask your surgeon at www.recoverquicklyfromsurgery.com/questions
_____

Choose all appropriate protocols
_____

CHAPTER 15

PRACTICAL MATTERS

It is often in the darkest skies that we see the brightest stars.

—Richard Evans

If you will be bedridden in the hospital or at home, it is important to be well prepared for your surgery. Even if your procedure is a minor one, check through the list below for those items that may be applicable to you.

1. **Transportation.** Arrange for a ride to and from the hospital in advance with family or helpers. It might be a good idea to have a backup plan.

2. **Hospital Essentials.** If you are staying overnight or longer, anticipate essentials such as toothbrush, hairbrush, make-up or any other necessary comfort items.

3. **Clothes.** Do laundry ahead of time and put clean linens on your bed. Put out clothes that you will want to wear, so that you do not have to exert yourself opening drawers or reaching for items. Plan the clothes that you will wear home after being released from surgery. You will probably want to wear loose clothing over the delicate area of operation.

4. **Insurance Coverage.** Check with your insurance company about the extent of your policy's coverage for surgery, anesthesia and any necessary follow-up. Make sure that your surgery is covered and authorized.

5. **Homeopathic Remedies.** Bring your homeopathic remedies to accelerate your recovery in the hospital.

6. **Food.** Have someone organize food for you if you will be unable to cook. Plan to have friends make food in shifts and deliver it to you on particular days. Prepare food and freeze meals that are easy to heat.

7. **Prescriptions.** Your surgeon will give you the prescriptions ahead of time. Plan to get prescription medicines filled and acquire other necessities before your surgery to have them ready for your home care.

8. **Home Safety.** Check home for tripping hazards such as electrical cords, throw rugs, toys and furniture. Make sure you have a non-slip surface in your tub and shower. Install nightlights to light your way to the bathroom at night. Make sure handrails on stairs are secure.

9. **Cell Phone.** It can be extremely draining to be on the phone in the first few days of recovery while you are recovering. Once you feel better, have a cordless or cell phone nearby.

10. **Pets.** If you have pets that are demanding or that jump on you, you may want to board them for a few days. If they remain at home, make sure that there is someone to feed and walk them if you are bedridden. Think through all of their needs before surgery.

11. **At Home Physical Supports.** If required, rent a hospital bed and have it delivered before you arrive home. Acquire any of these necessary items as well: walker, crutches, wheelchair, bandages, orthopedic supports, icing machines and bedpan.

12. **Support.** Anticipate any support or visitations from friends you might need—before your surgery. If you belong to a church,

synagogue or community organization, be sure to ask for prayers and good wishes from your community.

13. **"Point Person"**. If you having a serious procedure, ask a friend to be in charge of informing others about your progress. Prepare an email list of friends and family and forward it to them.

14. **Mail**. If bedridden, arrange to have someone bring in your mail and newspapers.

15. **Allow Time to Heal**. Allow yourself plenty of time after surgery with no commitments. Do not schedule any events, in case you do not feel as well as you anticipate. Stock up on good videos, books and magazines to keep you occupied and to take your mind off any pain or boredom you may experience.

16. **Legal Matters**. Make sure you have all your legal documents such as a living trust, a will, healthcare directive and power of attorney in order.

17. **Bills Paid in Advance**. To alleviate any future stress, try to pay all bills in advance.

18. **Tie Up Loose Ends At Work**. If possible, get someone to cover your work responsibilities for your expected recovery time, and complete all business transactions before your surgery. It will give you the peace of mind you will need.

! TAKE ACTION

Download checklist of protocols from www. recoverquicklyfromsurgery.com and prepare to recovery quickly!

CHAPTER 16

THE DAY OF YOUR SURGERY

I learned that courage was not the absence of fear,
but the triumph over it. The brave man is not he who
does not feel afraid, but he who conquers that fear.

—Nelson Mandela

PRE-ADMITTANCE

Your surgeon will have ordered any necessary tests prior to the day of surgery to rule out any issues that may prohibit surgery. He or she will also give you a list of instructions specific for your procedure.

HOSPITAL ADMITTANCE: THE ROUTINE

Once admitted, you will be asked to sign a consent form giving your permission for surgery to go as scheduled. This form indicates that you know what the surgery is for and that you understand the risks, benefits and alternative treatments. You will then be asked to change into a hospital gown, and the details of the operation will be explained. There may be final, routine preparations made and further tests or medications given to you while you wait to go into the surgical waiting area. You may meet your anesthesiologist and other nurses or physicians who will assist you and explain the procedure to you, as well as answer questions.

You will then be taken into the operating room, where you may be given anesthesia to allow you to undergo the operation with no pain. You may also be connected to a drip of nutrients, antibiotics or other medications.

Once your surgery is completed, you will be admitted to a recovery room where the attending nurse will administer tests to determine your lung capacity. They may provide support stockings to assist in preventing blood clots from forming. You will be asked about your pain levels, and, your pain medication will be adjusted as needed.

Once you have stabilized, you will be transferred to a hospital room where you may stay for as little as a few hours or as long as weeks, depending on the complexity of your surgical procedure.

YOUR HOSPITAL STAY

- If you have not already done so, inform your physician and staff of any medications, allergies or issues with taking medications in the past.

- You may be asked to receive a flu or pneumonia vaccination. Discuss this with your physician if you have issues with getting flu shots.

- Once in your room, inform your doctor, nurse or nutritionist if you wish to continue to follow the Recover Quickly Diet or anti-inflammatory diet in the hospital. They can arrange a diet of vegetables and light proteins with no sugar or desserts.

- Always ask for assistance in getting out of bed until you are sure that you are steady on your feet.

- Keep your nurses informed if pain levels rise or if swelling increases in any area of the body. Ask to have the call button always within reach. Ask questions if you are confused about treatment or hospital protocols.

- Make sure your advocate or family reports any negative

changes in your condition.

- Have family members wash their hands before they come and see you. Advise anyone with a cold to refrain from visiting until they are well.

- If you have a respiratory issue, use tissues rather than your hands if you must sneeze or cough.

POST-SURGICAL RECOVERY

You will want to follow your surgeon's instructions for your recovery once you are home. This will include proper wound care, taking the correct medication dosage, as well as getting ample rest.

In addition, your recovery will be greatly accelerated by maintaining the Recovery Quickly Diet and supplement protocols. You may feel especially tired from the anesthesia and may want to use the homeopathic remedies to gently detoxify it from your system.

QUESTIONS FOR YOUR SURGEON AFTER YOUR SURGERY

- Who should I call if I have any concerns once I'm home? May I have your cell number?

- When can I use the bathroom on my own?

- What activities should be avoided?

- How much pain, bruising or swelling is expected and for how long?

- When and where will any stitches be removed?

- Do I need a follow-up appointment? If so, when will this be?

- When can I go back to work? Sports? Household chores? Lifting?

It is important to resist doing too much once you are feeling better. Remember, there are treatments to assist in your healing process, such as acupuncture, chiropractic, physical therapy and laser therapy. Use your mind-body techniques to supercharge the healing process and to keep positive about your recovery. To the best of your ability, enjoy the recovery process – this positive attitude will greatly accelerate your healing time.

DISCHARGE FROM THE HOSPITAL

Make sure you or your advocate is clear about your discharge instructions. Before you leave the hospital, you may have an appointment with a physical therapist for exercises to aid in your recovery. You may also have a consultation and/or be given handouts about wound care, use of pain medication and icing. You may also be given necessary equipment such as crutches, supports, or machines to assist with range of motion or icing.

Each hospital will have its own policy and arrangements for discharging patients. Your level of health and the nature of your surgery will determine when you are discharged and the level of support you'll need upon returning home.

MEDICAL EMERGENCIES

Your hospital and surgeon may give you a list of negative reactions or symptoms that may indicate a surgical complication has occurred. Call 911 or your surgeon immediately if any of these symptoms arise:

- spitting up blood

- rapid or pounding heart rate

- heart or chest pain

- difficulty breathing

- redness, tenderness, swelling or heat in your calves or other areas (possibly indicating blood clots)

164

- feeling faint

Call your surgeon immediately if any of these symptoms develop:

- skin rashes, itching or red streaking under the skin
- broken stiches or wounds splitting open
- rapid heart rate or dizziness
- a fever of 100 degrees or higher
- sweating, chills or shaking
- swelling in your legs
- increased redness, pain or tenderness around the incision
- a yellowish, foul smelling discharge from the wound
- a lingering tiredness that does not subside
- nausea, vomiting, diarrhea or abdominal cramps
- numbness or tingling around the incision
- uncontrolled bleeding from anywhere
- black or tarry stools
- blood in urine, blood in your stool or blood in your vomit

! TAKE ACTION

Download the appropriate questions to ask your surgeon at www.recoverquicklyfromsurgery.com/questions

Prepare to recover quickly!

CHAPTER 17
HINDSIGHT

An ounce of prevention is worth a pound of cure.

—Henry de Bracton

One of the most important lessons gained from any surgical experience may be to realize how you acquired your condition or injury. Some physicians will review with their patients the probable cause of their injuries or illness and this awareness can help prevent the return of that condition. Sometimes, such as in the case of an accident, the injury was simply beyond anyone's control.

THE POWER OF INSIGHT

If you have not determined what caused your condition or injury, here are some questions that you may ask your surgeon.

- What caused my condition?

- How could I have prevented it?

- How can I prevent re-injury or a reoccurrence?

- Are there any nutritional factors that can optimize my healing or prevent a reoccurrence?

- Are there any orthopedic supports that could have prevented this injury or help me recover?

- Am I in danger of a reoccurrence?

- Has stress contributed to this condition?

If your surgeon does not have the answers to these questions, perhaps another healthcare professional might.

THE ROLE OF GENETICS

Family genetics and habits such as poor diet and lack of exercise may play a role in your condition. Children are prone to experience similar health issues as their relatives at similar points in their lives – unless they significantly change causative lifestyles.

When patients express fears about developing family health issues, I ask if smoking, excessive drinking, poor diet or a lack of exercise could have contributed to their family's health issues. Many patients fail to recognize the connection between health and lifestyle, and do not understand they have the ability to make the necessary changes for prevention.

Once someone makes the connection, it is up to them to initiate changes that will lead to a healthy lifestyle. If making that change by themselves seems difficult, a healthcare practitioner such as a holistic chiropractor, an acupuncturist, a naturopath or life coach will be more than willing to offer advice and follow through with the patient.

Hindsight can be a costly way of learning. Foresight requires more effort, but in the long run prevents health issues from developing.

Even after your surgery, do not discontinue your relationship with your complementary medicine practitioner. They are trained in the *prevention* of health issues by focusing on maintaining a healthy lifestyle. They are required to update their education yearly. Scientists and the medical profession continue to provide research backing many of the health-style practices that have been utilized in complementary medicine for years.

VIEW YOUR SURGICAL EXPERIENCE AS A CATALYST

Over the years, I have noticed that those patients who discovered some meaning or lesson from their surgical experience or their illness or condition itself, had an easier time with their recovery process. In these cases, the surgical experience became more about the lesson learned than the surgery itself.

If you wish to glean a new life lesson, examine your former lifestyle, exercise habits, diet, work, stress levels and approach to life. Create more balance in your life so as to avoid future health issues. Focus on caring for yourself in a new way to prevent a future health crisis.

Remember: *you only have one body.* Allow your surgery to serve as a catalyst for a new, healthier and more exciting life. Become more educated about your health options. From now on, proactively participate in your health with your new holistic health care practitioner at your side. Allow them to become an *accountability coach* that can create a plan with you to change old habits, begin a new exercise regime and utilize nutritional supplements that can detoxify and rebuild your system. This change in your former habits will lead to a more youthful, vibrant lifestyle. And therein lies the silver lining from your surgery. Long may you live.

ENDNOTES

1. Thomas Bodenheimer, MD; Kate Lorig, RN, DrPH; Halsted Holman,MD; Kevin Grumbach, MD; Patient Self-management of Chronic Disease in Primary Care ; Innovations in Primary Care ; JAMA. 2002; 288(19): 2469-2475l,November 20, 2002 ; Giraudet-Le Quintrec, Janine-Sophie MD; Coste, Joël MD, PhD; Vastel, Laurent MD; Pacault, Véronique MD; Jeanne, Luc MD et al; Positive Effect of Patient Education for Hip Surgery: A Randomized Trial; *Clinical Orthopaedics percent Related Research*: September 2003 - Volume 414 - Issue - pp 112-120; Judith H. Hibbard; , Jessica Greene; Valerie Overton; Patients With Lower Activation Associated With Higher Costs; Delivery Systems Should Know Their Patients' Scores 10.1377/hlthaff.2012.1064, Health Affairs; February 2013 vol. 32 no. 2 216-222

2. National Center for Complementary and Alternative Medicine (NCCAM) and the National Center for Health Statistics; December 2008, as cited at http://nccam. nih.gov/news/camstats/2007/camsurvey_fs1.htm; Ernst E (September 2003). "Obstacles to research in complementary and alternative medicine". *The Medical Journal of Australia* 179 (6): 279–80. PMID 12964907; Barnes PM, Powell-Griner E, McFann K, Nahin RL (May 2004). "Complementary and alternative medicine use among adults: United States, 2002". *Advance Data* (343): 1–19. PMID 15188733.

3. Topp R, Swank AM, Quesada PM, et al, The effect of prehabilitation exercise on strength and functioning after total knee arthroplasty. PM& Journal.2009 Aug;1(8):729

4. Rizzo, Terrie Heinrich, "Prehab for Surgery", as cited in *Arthritis Today*, at http://www.arthritistoday.org/treatments/surgery/prehab-for-surgery.php

5. Brown K, Swank AM, Quesada PM, Nyland J, Malkani A, Topp R, Prehabilitation versus usual care before total knee arthroplasty: A case report comparing outcomes within the same individual, *Physiotherapy Theory and Practice*. 2010 Aug; 26(6):399-407.

6. Rooks, D. Arthritis percent Rheumatism, Oct. 15, 2006; vol 55: pp 700-708 as cited in *CBS News Healthwatch*, Exercise Before Joint Replacement February 11, 2009 at http://www.cbsnews.com/stories/2006/09/29/health/webmd/main2053669.shtml?source=related_story

7. Brouziyne M, Molinaro C. "Mental imagery combined with physical practice of approach shots for golf beginners." *Perceptual and Motor Skills.* 2005 Aug;101(1):203-11.

8. Mark A. Williams, William L. Haskell, Philip A. Ades, Ezra A. Amsterdam, Vera Bittner, Barry A. Franklin, Meg Gulanick, Susan T. Laing, and Kerry J. Stewart; Resistance Exercise in Individuals With and Without Cardiovascular Disease: 2007 Update. A Scientific Statement From the American Heart Association Council on Clinical Cardiology and Council on Nutrition, Physical Activity, and Metabolism." Circulation, Published online before print July 16, 2007, doi:10.1161/CIRCULATIONAHA.107.185214 ; Hayden JA, van Tulder MW, Tomlinson G. Systematic review: strategies for using exercise therapy to improve outcomes in chronic low back pain. *Annals of Internal Medicine.* 2005;142(9):776-785; Life Stages With Ulcerative Colitis ; *Webmd*: Living Well With Ulcerative Colitis Tips for living with UC at every life stage: How Exercise Can Help Ulcerative Colitis as cited at http://www.webmd.com/ibd-crohns-disease/ulcerative-colitis-10/default.htm

9. Shirley Tellles, B. Hanumanthaih, R. Nagarathna, and H. R. Nagendra;Vivekananda, Improvement in Static Motor Performance Following Yogic Training of School Children; *Kendra Yoga Research Foundation*, Bangalore, India. March 22. 1993

10. Karen J. Sherman, PhD, MPH; Daniel C. Cherkin, PhD; Robert D. Wellman, MS; Andrea J. Cook, PhD; Rene J. Hawkes, BS; Kristin Delaney, MPH; Richard A. Deyo, MD, MPH; A Randomized Trial Comparing Yoga, Stretching, and a Self-care Book for Chronic Low Back Pain; *Archives of Internal Medicine* (Now *JAMA*). 2011;171(22):2019-2026. doi:10.1001/archinternmed.2011.524

11. Yoga for Anxiety and Depression, Harvard Medical Health Letter, April 2009 as cited at http://www.health.harvard.edu/newsletters/Harvard_Mental_Health_Letter/2009/April/Yoga-for-anxiety-and-depression

12. Wang C, Schmid CH, Hibberd PL, Kalish, et al, Tai Chi is effective in treating knee osteoarthritis: a randomized controlled trial; Arthritis and Rheumatism. 2009 Nov 15;61(11):1545-53.

---

13. Abdulaziz Al-Rasheed, Khalid Almas, George E. Romanos and Khalid Al-Hezaimi. (2011) Effect of Cigarette Smoking on the Clinical Outcomes of Periodontal Surgical Procedures. *The American Journal of the Medical Sciences*1; Online publication date: 1-Jul-2011 Antonios Mavropoulos, Pål Brodin, Cassiano Kuchenbecker Rösing, Anne Merete Aass and Harald Aars. (2007) Gingival Blood Flow in Periodontitis Patients Before and After Periodontal Surgery Assessed in Smokers and Non-Smokers. *Journal of Periodontology* 78:9, 1774-1782; Online publication date: 1-Sep-2007;Castillo, Renan C. MSc*; Bosse, Michael J. MD†; MacKenzie, Ellen J. PhD*; Patterson, Brendan M. MD‡; the LEAP Study Group; Impact of Smoking on Fracture Healing and Risk of Complications in Limb-Threatening Open Tibia Fractures; *Journal of Orthopaedic Trauma*; March 2005, Vol 19, Issue 3- pp 151-157

---

14. Health Watch—Heal Faster, Southwestern Medical Center as cited at http://www. utsouthwestern.edu/utsw/cda/dept16498/files/145519.html, January 2004

---

15. Effect of Smoking Cessation Intervention on Results of Acute Fracture Surgery: A Randomized Controlled Trial, Journal of Bone and Joint Surgery, *Journal of Bone and Joint Surgery*, Jun 2010; 92: 1335 – 1342

---

16. Environmental Protection Agency. Respiratory Health Effects of Passive Smoking: Lung Cancer and Other Disorders. Washington, DC: *Environmental Protection Agency*; 1992. (Report # EPA/600/6-90/006F) Accessed at: http://cfpub2. epa.gov/ncea/cfm/recordisplay.cfm?deid=2835 on November 3, 2010; U.S. Department of Health and Human Services. The Health Consequences of Involuntary Exposure to Tobacco Smoke: *A Report of the Surgeon General. Washington, DC: Department of Health and Human Services*; 2006. Accessed at www.surgeongeneral.gov/library/secondhandsmoke/ on November 2, 2010

---

17. as cited at http://www.wisegeek.org/is-there-caffeine-in-chocolate.htm

---

18. Effects of Ethanol on Cytokine Production After Surgery in a Murine Model of Gram-Negative Pneumonia; Alcoholism: *Clinical and Experimental Research*

32 (2), 331–338 and cited at Jha, Alok, "Doctors warn of alcohol risk to patients facing surgery", *The Guardian* as cited at http://www.guardian.co.uk/science/2008/feb/04/medicalresearch.drugsandalcohol February 3, 2008.

19. Crumley, A. B. C., McMillan, M. McKernan, et al, "Evaluation of an Inflammation-Based Prognostic Score (GPS) in Patients with Inoperable Gastrooesophageal Cancer", *British Journal of Cancer*, 94, no.5 (2006):637-41; Al Murri, A. M., J. M. S Bartlett, P.A. Canney, et al, "Evaluation of an Inflammation-Based Prognostic Score (GPS) in Patients with Metastatic Breast Cancer", *British Journal of Cancer* 94, no.2, (2006): 227-30

20. Provost, D., A. Gruber, P. Lebailly, et al. "Brain Tumors and Exposure to Pesticides: A case-Control Study in Southwestern France", *Occupational and Environmental Medicine*, 2007

21. Leffers H, Naesby M, Vendelbo B, et al. (2001). Oestrogenic potencies of zeranol, oestradiol, diethylstilbestrol, bisphenol-A and genistein: Implications for exposure assessment of potential endocrine disrupters. *Human Reproduction*, 16:1037-1045.

22. Gunter, M. J., et al, "Insulin, Insulin-Like Growth Factor-I, and Risk of Breast Cancer in Post menopausal Women", *Journal of the National Cancer Institute* 101, (2009): 48-60

23. Nancy Appleton, Nancy, Ph.D."146 Reasons Why Sugar Is Ruining Your Health" *Rheumatic.org* as cited at http://nancyappleton.com/141-reasons-sugar-ruins-your-health/

24. Beier, R. C. Natural pesticides and bioactive components in foods. *Reviews of Environmental and Contamination Toxicology*. 1990; 113:47-137; Childers N.F. A relationship of arthritis to the Solanaceae (nightshades). *J Intern Acad Prev Med* 1979; 7:31-37

25."Mercury Levels in Commercial Fish and Shellfish" as cited at http://www.fda.gov/food/foodsafety/product-specific information/seafood/foodbornepathogenscontaminants/methylmercury/ucm115644.htm FDA , *US Food And Drug Administration*; (1990-2010)

26. Mao Shing Ni, Dr. Mao's Wellness Central: Four Best and Worst Foods for Blood

Pressure; Jun. 23, 2011; as cited on *Santa Monica Mirror*: www.smmirror.co
m/?ajax#mode=singlepercentview=32391

27. Hirofumi Tachibana, Kiyoshi Koga, Yoshinori Fujimura,percent Koji Yamada
"A Receptor For Green Tea Polyphenol EGCG", *Nature Structural percent
Molecular Biology* 11, 380 - 381 (2004) Published online: 14 March 2004;
Bursill C, Roach PD, Bottema CD, Pal S., "Green tea up regulates the low-
density lipoprotein receptor through the sterol-regulated element binding
Protein in HepG2 liver cells; *Journal of Agricultural and Food Chemistry*.
2001 Nov; 49(11):5639-45 and Shanafelt TD, Call TG, Zent CS, et al. Phase
I trial of daily oral Polyphenon E in patients with asymptomatic Rai stage 0
to II chronic lymphocytic leukemia. *Journal of Clinical Oncology*. 2009 Aug
10;27(23):3808-3814.

28. Mehta, K., P. Pantazis, T. McQueen, et al, "Antiproliferative Effect of Cucumin
(Diferuloylmethane) Against Human Breast Tumor Cell Lines"*Anti-Cancer
Drugs* 8, no.5 (1997) 470-81

29. Wagner M, Oehlmann J (2009): Endocrine disruptors in bottled mineral water:
Total estrogenic burden and migration from plastic bottles. *Environmental and.
Science and Pollution Research*; 16, 278-286.

30. Rahn H-D. Efficacy of hydrolytic enzymes in surgery. Presented at: Symposium
on Enzyme Therapy in Sports Injuries: XXIV FIMS *World Congress of Sport
Medicine*; May 29 1990; Amsterdam, The Netherlands; Vinzenz K. Treatment
of edema with hydrolytic enzymes in oral surgical procedures [translated from
German]. *Quintessenz*. 1991;42:1053-1064; Zuschlag JM. Double-blind
clinical study using certain proteolytic enzyme mixtures in karate fighters
[working paper]. In: *Mucos Pharma GmbH*(Germany). 1988;1-5; Rathgeber
WF. The use of proteolytic enzymes (chymoral) in sporting injuries. *South
African Medical Journal*. 1971; 45:181-183;

31. Pecking AP, Fevrier B, Wargon C, et al. Efficacy of Daflon 500 mg in the
treatment of lymphedema (secondary to conventional therapy of breast cancer).
Angiology. 1997;48:93-98 and Fassina A, Rubinacci A. Post-traumatic edema:
a controlled study into the activity of hydroxyethyl rutoside [translated from
Italian]. *Gazz Med Ital Arch Sci* . 1987;146:103-109 as cited at NYU Lagone
Medical Center at http://surgery.med.nyu.edu/content?ChunkIID=21452#ref17

32. Vinciguerra P, Camesasca FI, Ponzin D., "Use of Amino Acids in Refractive Surgery"; *Journal of Refractive Surgery*, 2002 May-Jun;18(3 Suppl):S374-7

33. Society of Homeopaths : What is Homeopathy? As cited at http://www. homeopathy-soh.org/about-homeopathy/what-is-homeopathy/

34. Kim LS, Axelrod LJ, Howard P, Buratovich N, Waters RF. "Efficacy of methylsulfonyl-methane (MSM) in osteoarthritis pain of the knee: a pilot clinical trial." *Osteoarthritis and Cartilage* 2006; 14:286

35. National Cancer Institute, "Human/Clinical Studies : Effect of Acupuncture on Immune Function; Effect of Acupuncture on Cancer Pain; Effect of Acupuncture on Cancer Treatment–related Side Effects"; as cited at http:// www.cancer.gov/cancertopics/pdq/cam/acupuncture/healthprofessional/ page5 June 2011; Harmon D, Gardiner J, Harrison R, et al. Acupressure and the prevention of nausea and vomiting after laparoscopy. *British Journal of Anaesethia*. 1999;82:387-390. ; Harmon D, Ryan M, Kelly A, et al. Acupressure and prevention of nausea and vomiting during and after spinal anaesthesia for caesarean section. *British Jouranl of Anaesethia*. 2000;84:463-467. ; Alkaissi A, Stalnert M, Kalman S. Effect and placebo effect of acupressure (P6) on nausea and vomiting after outpatient gynaecological surgery. *Acta Anaesthesiol Scand*. 1999;43:270-274.;Ho CM, Hseu SS, Tsai SK, et al. Effect of P-6 acupressure on prevention of nausea and vomiting after epidural morphine for post-cesarean section pain relief. *Acta Anaesthesiologica Scandinavica Foundation*. 1996;40:372-375.

36. *Duke Medicine News and Communications*, "Acupuncture Reduces Pain, Need for Opioids after Surgery" , cited at www.dukehealth.org/health_library/ news/10153, October 16, 2007

37. Wang, Shu-Ming; Gaal, D; Maranets, I, Kain, Z; et al; "Acupressure and Preoperative Parental Anxiety: A Pilot Study" Anesthesia and Analgesia, Sept 2005 and cited at University of California, UC Newsroom, "Acupressure Calms Children before Surgery" as cited at http://www.universityofcalifornia. edu/news/article/18670 09-30-08.

38. Depending on How Much and How Long, Light from Self-Luminous Tablet Computers Can Affect Evening Melatonin, Delaying Sleep; Lighting Research

Center; as cited at http://www.lrc.rpi.edu/resources/newsroom/pr_story.
asp?id=235; 8/21/2012

39. Davidson, R. J., J. Kabat-Zinn, J. Schumacher, et al.,"Alterations in Immune
and Brain Function produces by Mindfulness Meditation", *Psychosomatic
Medicine* 65, no.4 (2003): 564-570

40. E. Solberg et al, 'Meditation: a modulator of the immune response to physical
stress?', *British Journal of Sports Medicine*, vo. 29(4), pp255-257) 1995

41. Stress In America, *American Psychological Association*, Report 2010 as cited at
http://www.apa.org/news/press/releases/stress/key-findings.aspx

42. Moseley JB, et al. A controlled trial of arthroscopic surgery for osteoarthritis of
the knee. *New England Journal of Medicine.* July 11, 2002;347(2):81-88.

43. McCarthy, SC (McCarthy, SC); Lyons, AC (Lyons, AC); Weinman, J (Weinman,
J); Talbot, R (Talbot, R); Purnell, D (Purnell, D), "Do expectations influence
recovery from oral surgery? An illness representation approach." *Psychology
percent Health* Volume: 18 Issue: 1 Pages: 109-126; FEB 2003

44. Cole, D. C., Mondloch, M. V., Hogg-Johnson, S., percent Early Claimant
Cohort Prognostic Modelling Group. (2002). Listening to injured workers:
How recovery expectations predict outcomes--A prospective study. *Canadian
Medical Association Journal*, 166, 749 754.

45. Davis, Lerche Jeanie; Can Prayer Heal? Does prayer have the power to heal?
WebMD Feature; as cited at http://www.webmd.com/balance/features/can-
prayer-heal

46. Tusek, D; Church, James; Strong, Scott, et al; Guided Imagery; *Diseases of the
Colon percent Rectum* ; February 1997, Volume 40, Issue 2, pp 172-178
as cited at http://link.springer.com/journal/10350; Guided Imagery: Its use
in Heart Surgery and other Procedures, *Cleveland Clinic* as cited at http://
my.clevelandclinic.org/heart/prevention/stress/guided_imagery.aspx

47. Cassels, C.; Meditation Improves Endothelial Function in Metabolic
Syndrome;Pilot study may have implications for reducing cardiovascular risk
in African Americans. *Medscape Medical News*; March 18, 2011 as cited at

http://www.medscape.com/viewarticle/739296

48. Bennett, H. L., Benson, D. R., Kuiken, D. A. Preoperative Instructions for Decreased Bleeding During Spine Surgery. *Anesthesiology*, (1986)Vol. 65, A245.Devine, E. C; Effects of Psychoeducational Care for Adult Surgical Patients: A meta-analysis of 191 studies. *Patient Education and Counseling*, (1992). Vol. 19, pp. 129-142. Dreher, H. Mind-body interventions for surgery: evidence and exigency. *Advances in Mind-Body Medicine*, (1998). Vol. 14, pp. 207-222.

49. Sharma, H.; Meditation. Meditation. *Ohio State University Medical Center.* As cited at http://medicalcenter.osu.edu/patientcare/healthcare_services/services/?ID=1494

50. Meditation a Hit for Pain Management. NPR.org ; as cited at http://www.npr.org/templates/story/story.php?storyId=7654964. March 1, 2007.; Meditation May Help Brain Handle Pain. *Medscape Today*.; as cited at http://www.medscape.com/viewarticle/542553 ; Mind over matter: Meditation helps ease pain for some patients. CNN.com. September 4, 2000. http://archives.cnn.com/2000/HEALTH/alternative/09/04/meditation.pain.wmd/index.html ; National Pain Foundation: Using Complementary Therapy to Relieve Pain; as cited at http://www.nationalpainfoundation.org/mytreatment/News_Complementary.asp

51. Tusek, D; Church, James; Strong, Scott, et al; Guided Imagery; *Diseases of the Colon percent Rectum* ; February 1997, Volume 40, Issue 2, pp 172-178 as cited at http://link.springer.com/journal/10350; Guided Imagery: Its use in Heart Surgery and other Procedures, *Cleveland Clinic* as cited at http://my.clevelandclinic.org/heart/prevention/stress/guided_imagery.aspx

52. Gonzales EA, Ledesma RJ, McAllister DJ, Perry SM, Dyer CA, Maye JP; Effects of guided imagery on postoperative outcomes in patients undergoing same-day surgical procedures: a randomized, single-blind study. *American Association of Nurse Anesthetist Journal*, June 2010 ; 78(3):181-8.; Antall GF, Kresevic D.; The use of guided imagery to manage pain in an elderly orthopaedic population. *Orthopeadic Nursing*, 2004 Sep-Oct; 23(5):335-40.; Halpin LS, Speir AM, CapoBianco P, Barnett SD; Guided imagery in Cardiac Surgery; *Outcomes Management.* 2002 Jul-Sep;6(3):132-7

53. Ranganathan VK, Siemionow V, Liu JZ, Sahgal V, Yue GH ;From mental power to muscle power--gaining strength by using the mind; *Neuropsychologia*. 2004;42(7):944-56.; Reiser M, Büsch D, Munzert J.; Strength gains by motor imagery with different ratios of physical to mental practice; Frontiers in Psychology. 2011;2:194. Epub 2011 Aug 19.

54. Phend, C,; Hypnosis Before Surgery Dulls Pain Later; *MedPage Today*

August 28, 2007 citing Montgomery GH, et al "A Randomized Clinical Trial of a Brief Hypnosis Intervention to Control Side Effects in Breast Surgery Patients" *Journal of National Cancer Institute* 2007; 99: 1304-12 and Spiegel D "The Mind Prepared: Hypnosis in Surgery" *Journal of National Cancer Institute* 2007; 99: 1280-81.

55. Cromie, W.; Hypnosis Helps Healing: Surgical Wounds Mend Faster; *Harvard Gazette*, May 2003 as cited at http://news.harvard.edu/gazette/2003/05.08/01-hypnosis.html

56. American Cancer Society citing a NIH Report as cited at http://www.cancer.org/treatment/treatmentsandsideeffects/complementaryandalternativemedicine/mindbodyandspirit/hypnosis; Richardson J, Smith JE, McCall G, Pilkington K. Hypnosis for procedure-related pain and distress in pediatric cancer patients: a systematic review of effectiveness and methodology related to hypnosis interventions. *Journal of Pain Symptom Management*. 2006;31:70-84.

57. Giraudet-Le Quintrec, Janine-Sophie MD, et al, Positive Effect of Patient Education for Hip Surgery: A Randomized Trial , *Clinical Orthopaedics percent Related Research*: September 2003 - Volume 414 - Issue - pp 112-120

58. About Ambien, Ambien Addiction Treatment, as cited at http://www.ambien-addiction-treatment.com/category/about-ambien May 10, 2012; Stimson, Daniel, Ph.D, Resolvins' May Help Resolve Chronic Inflammatory Pain, *National Institute of Neurologiccal Disorders and Strokes*, as cited on http://www.ninds.nih.gov/news_and_events/news_articles/Resolvins_Chronic_Pain.htm Sept 17, 2010

59. Dusek, Jeffery A. PhD; Finch, Michael PhD†; Plotnikoff, Gregory MD, MTS, FACP‡; Knutson, Lori RN, BSN, HN-BC§; The Impact of Integrative

Medicine on Pain Management in a Tertiary Care Hospital; *Journal of Patient Safety*: March 2010 - Volume 6 - Issue 1 - pp 48-51

60. Mimi M. Y. Tse, M. F. Chan, and Iris F. F. Benzie; The Effect of Music Therapy on Postoperative Pain, Heart Rate, Systolic Blood Pressure and Analgesic Use Following Nasal Surgery; *Journal of Pain and Palliative Care Pharmacotherapy* 2005, Vol. 19, No. 3 : Pages 21-29 ; Randomized clinical trial examining the effect of music therapy in stress response to day surgery, *British Journal of Surgery*; Vol 94, issue 8 , pages 943–947, August 2007; WebMD Pain Management Health Center; Pain managemen: drug tolerance and addiction. As cited on http://www.webmd.com/pain-management/guide/drug-tolerance-addiction. Edited by Brunilda Nazario, MD on November 01, 2007

61. St. Joseph's Hospital and Medical Center, Slow breathing reduces pain; ScienceDaily. (2010, January 20); Zautra AJ, Fasman R et al; The effects of slow breathing on affective responses to pain stimuli: an experimental study as cited at http://www.ncbi.nlm.nih.gov/pubmed/20079569?itool=EntrezSystem2. PEntrez.Pubmed.Pubmed_ResultsPanel.Pubmed_RVDocSum&ordinalpos=1

62. Giovanna Delogu, MD; Sonia Moretti, MD; Giuseppe Famularo, MD; Sonia Marcellini, MD; Gino Santini, PhD; Adriana Antonucci, MD; Maurizio Marandola, MD; Luciano Signore, MD; A Mitochondrial Perturbations and Oxidant Stress in Lymphocytes From Patients Undergoing Surgery and General Anesthesia; *Archives of Surgery*. 2001;136:1190-1196

Printed in Great Britain
by Amazon